MARINATED GODDESS
SIMPLE AND SOULFUL

Summer Grilling and Outdoor Recipes

Copyright

MARINATED GODDESS
SIMPLE AND SOULFUL
Summer Grilling and Outdoor Recipes

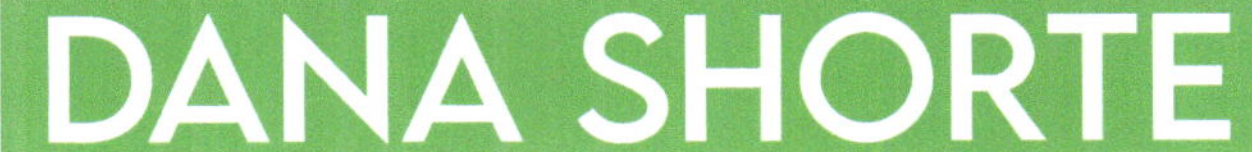

Disclaimer

Dana Shorte or any of her family members or affiliates are not responsible for your outcome of any recipe found in this book. There are a number of factors that could contribute to you not achieving the desired result when preparing any recipe. Some of those can include: the ingredients and brands of ingredients, your ingredient substitutions, skipping steps, combining steps, completing steps in a different order or altering the recipe, the equipment used, my possible errors/typos, or the reader's individual cooking ability.
My goal is your success with the recipes. I hope it comes out exactly as you hope it will, but sometimes it may not. I hope you'll always feel free to email me with a question so I can do my best to help.

Dedication

This first one is for my "Little Village" who helped me grow wings to fly, my forever Lovebug and my Earth Angel who gave me sight beyond sight.

TABLE OF CONTENTS

AUTHOR BIO

I worked in finance for the majority of my career as an executive and personal Assistant in Manhattan, NY. I loved what I did and I had a deep hunger in my belly to prove myself, provide for my family and to get ahead in corporate America. And then Covid-19 came out of nowhere and knocked the whole world on our asses!! Since we had to spend more time indoors, slow down and spend more quality time with family.I began my love affair with food. I learned how to cook as a teenager from watching my grandmother in the kitchen growing up but because I was always busy with work before, I never really had a lot of time to do it before the pandemic hit or if I did, I always felt rushed. During my time spent at home, I had free time to have fun with and be playful with food, create flavorful marinades and be daring with my grill. I choose my zestiest, healthiest, sauciest Summertime favorites to share in this sassy little cookbook. I hope you enjoy and share your experiences with me on social media.

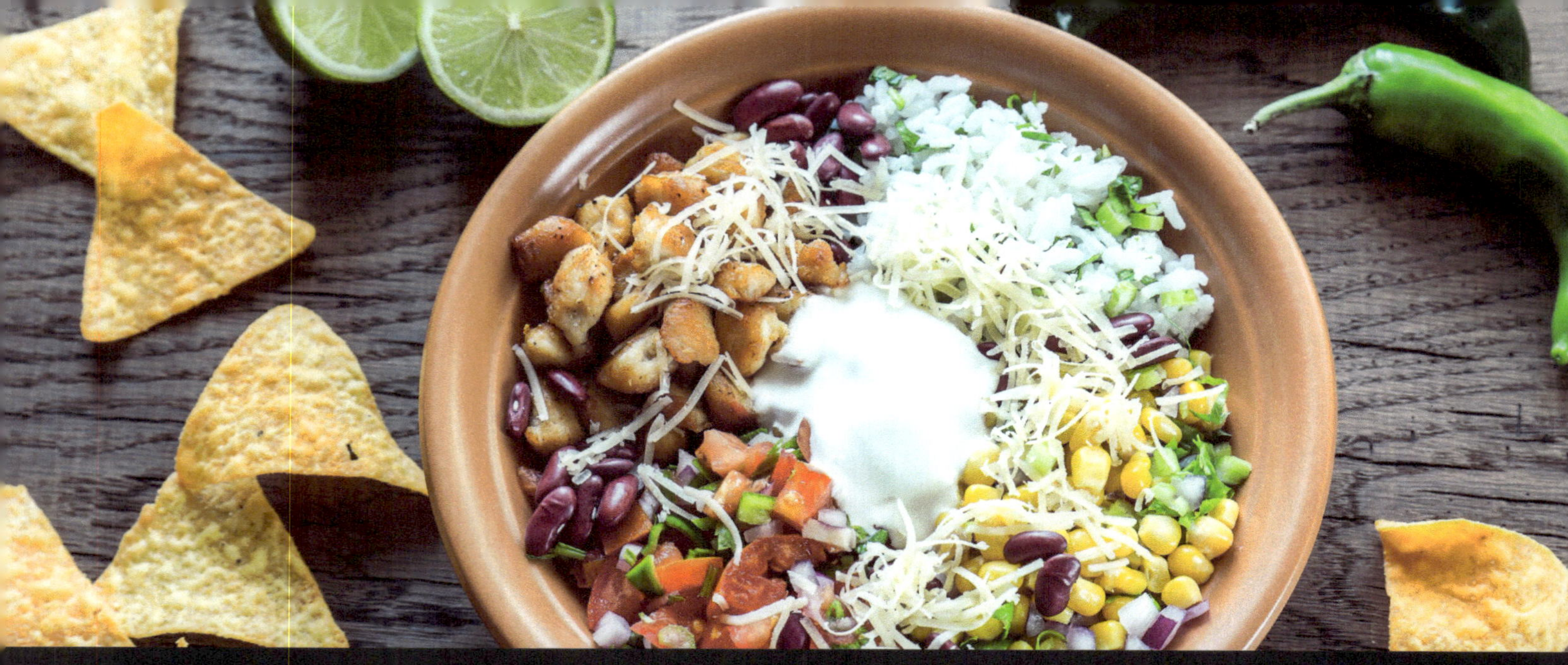

CHIPOTLE CHICKEN SALAD

<table>
<tr><th>Ingredients</th><th>Preparation Time
15 min</th><th>Cooking Time
20 min</th><th>Servings
4</th></tr>
</table>

Ingredients

- 2 boneless, skinless chicken breasts
- 1 tablespoon chipotle powder
- Salt and pepper to taste
- 8 cups mixed salad greens
- 1 cup cherry tomatoes, halved
- 1 avocado, sliced
- 1/4 cup low-fat ranch dressing

Directions

1. Preheat the grill to medium heat.
2. Season the chicken breasts with chipotle powder, salt, and pepper.
3. Grill the chicken for 10 minutes on each side or until cooked through. Let it rest for 5 mins, then slice.
4. Divide the salad greens, tomatoes, and avocado among four plates. Top with sliced chicken.
5. Drizzle each salad with 1 tablespoon of ranch dressing.

Nutrition Information

Calories: 300 , Total Fat: 14g , Total Carbohydrates: 10g , Fiber: 6g , Protein: 32g

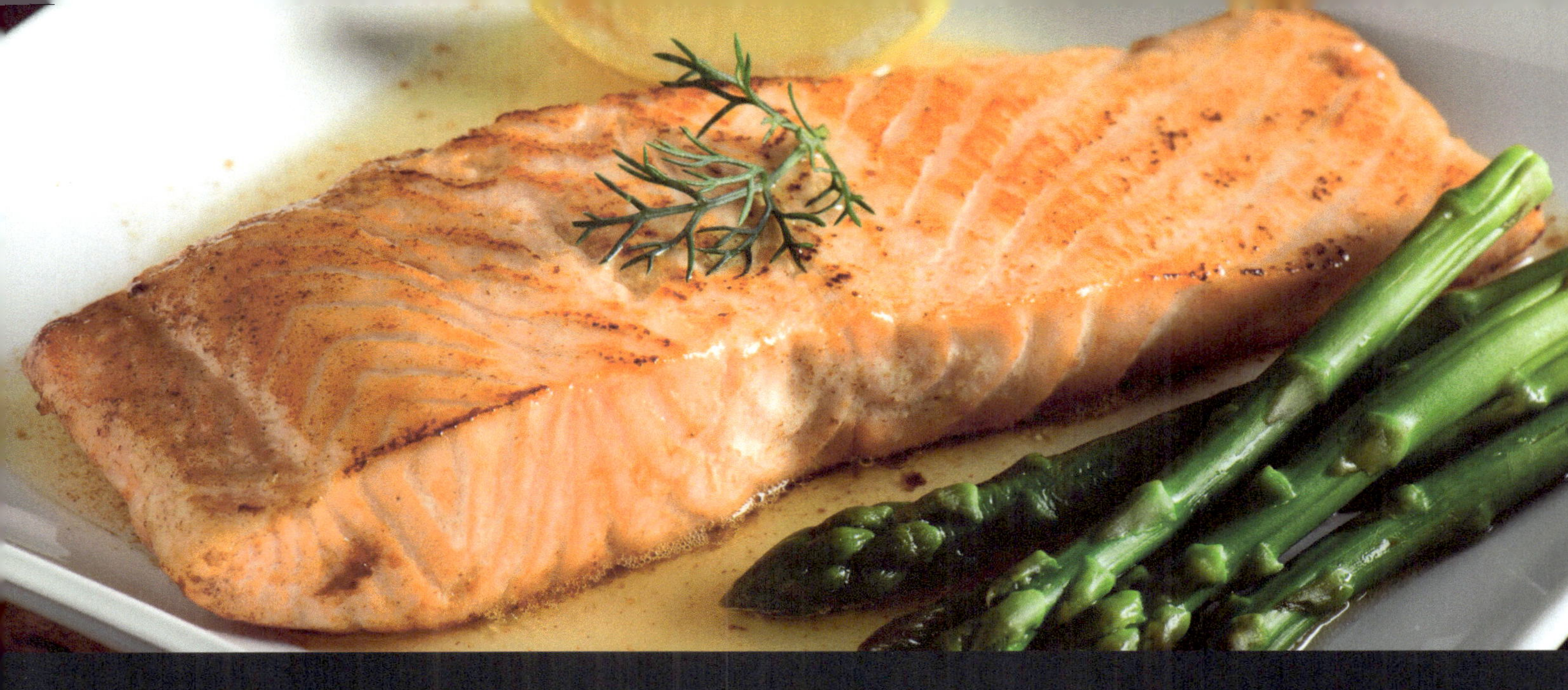

HERB-GRILLED SALMON

Ingredients

Preparation Time	Cooking Time	Servings
15 min	15 min	4

- 4 salmon fillets
- 2 tablespoons olive oil
- 1 tablespoon lemon juice
- 1 tablespoon mixed herbs (thyme, dill, parsley)
- Salt and pepper to taste

Directions

1. Preheat the grill to medium heat.
2. Mix olive oil, lemon juice, herbs, salt, and pepper in a bowl.
3. Brush the salmon fillets with the herb blending.
4. Grill for 6-8 minutes on each side until cooked to the desired doneness.

Nutrition Information

Calories: 310 , Total Fat: 20g , Total Carbohydrates: 1g , Fiber: 0g , Protein: 31g

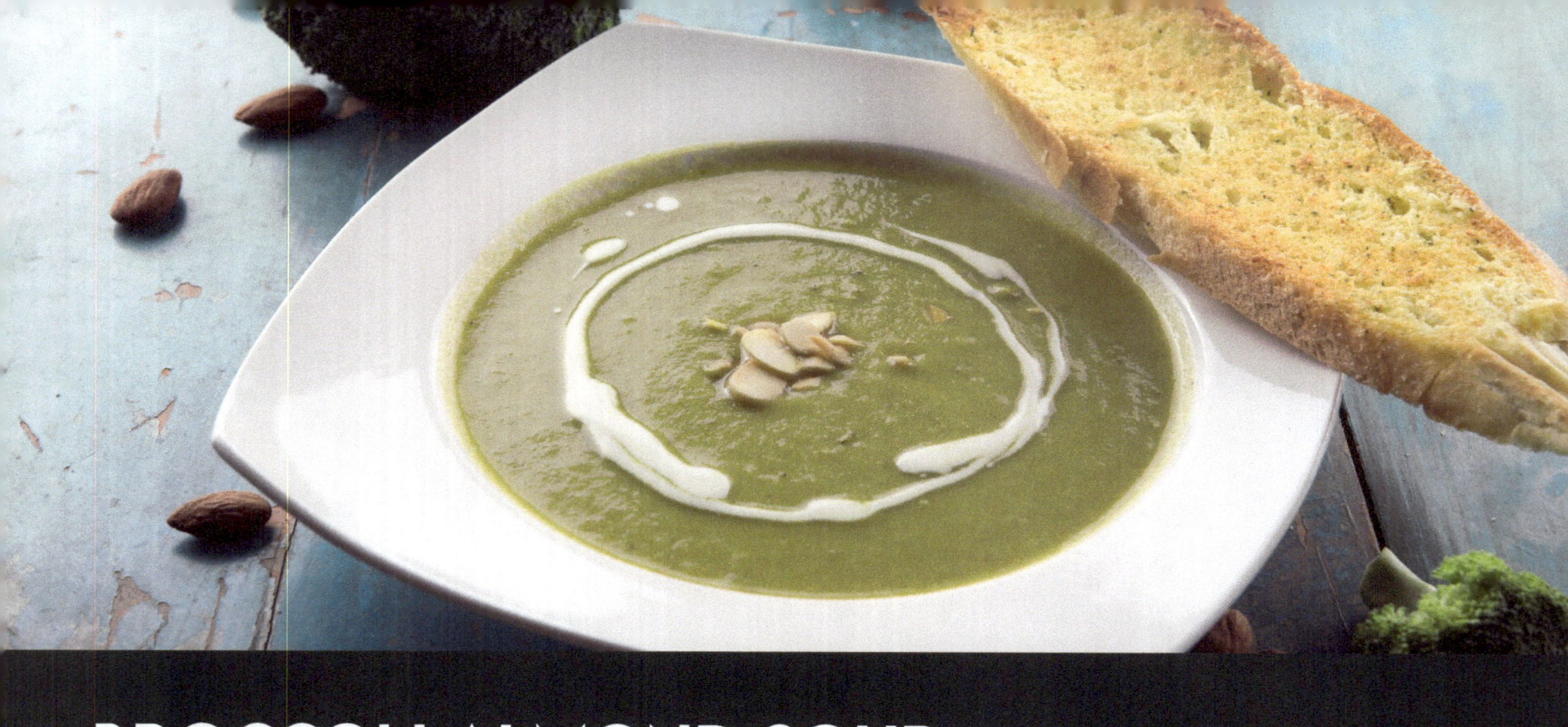

BROCCOLI ALMOND SOUP

Ingredients

Preparation Time	Cooking Time	Servings
10 min	20 min	4

- 1 tablespoon olive oil
- 1 onion, chopped
- 2 cloves garlic, minced
- 4 cups broccoli florets
- 4 cups vegetable broth
- 1/2 cup almond milk
- Salt and pepper to taste

Directions

1. Medium-heat olive oil in a saucepan. Cook onion and garlic till tender.
2. Add broccoli and vegetable broth. Set to a boil, then simmer for 10 to 15 minutes until the broccoli is softened.
3. Combine the soup with an immersion blender until smooth.
4. Stir in almond milk and season with salt and pepper.

Nutrition Information

Calories: 150 , Total Fat: 7g , Total Carbohydrates: 18g , Fiber: 5g , Protein: 5g

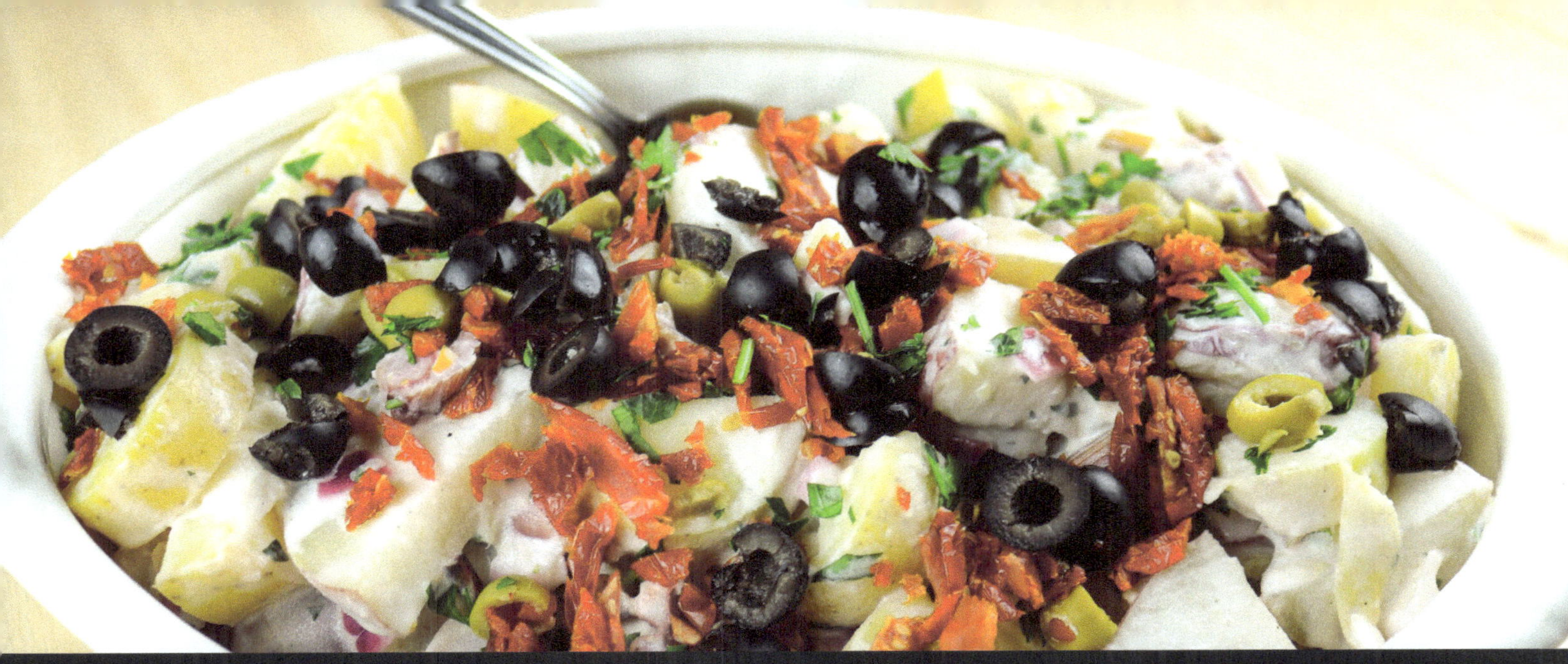

TANGY GREEK SALAD

Preparation Time	Cooking Time	Servings
15 min	0 min	4

Ingredients

- 4 cups romaine lettuce, chopped
- 1 cucumber, diced
- 1 cup cherry tomatoes, halved
- 1/2 cup Kalamata olives
- 1/2 cup feta cheese, crumbled
- 1/4 cup red wine vinegar
- 1/2 cup olive oil
- Salt and pepper to taste

Directions

1. Combine lettuce, cucumber, tomatoes, olives, and feta in a large bowl.
2. Whisk together red wine vinegar, olive oil, salt, and pepper in a small bowl.
3. Drizzle the dressing over the salad just prior serving.

Nutrition Information

Calories: 290 , Total Fat: 25g , Total Carbohydrates: 10g , Fiber: 3g , Protein: 5g

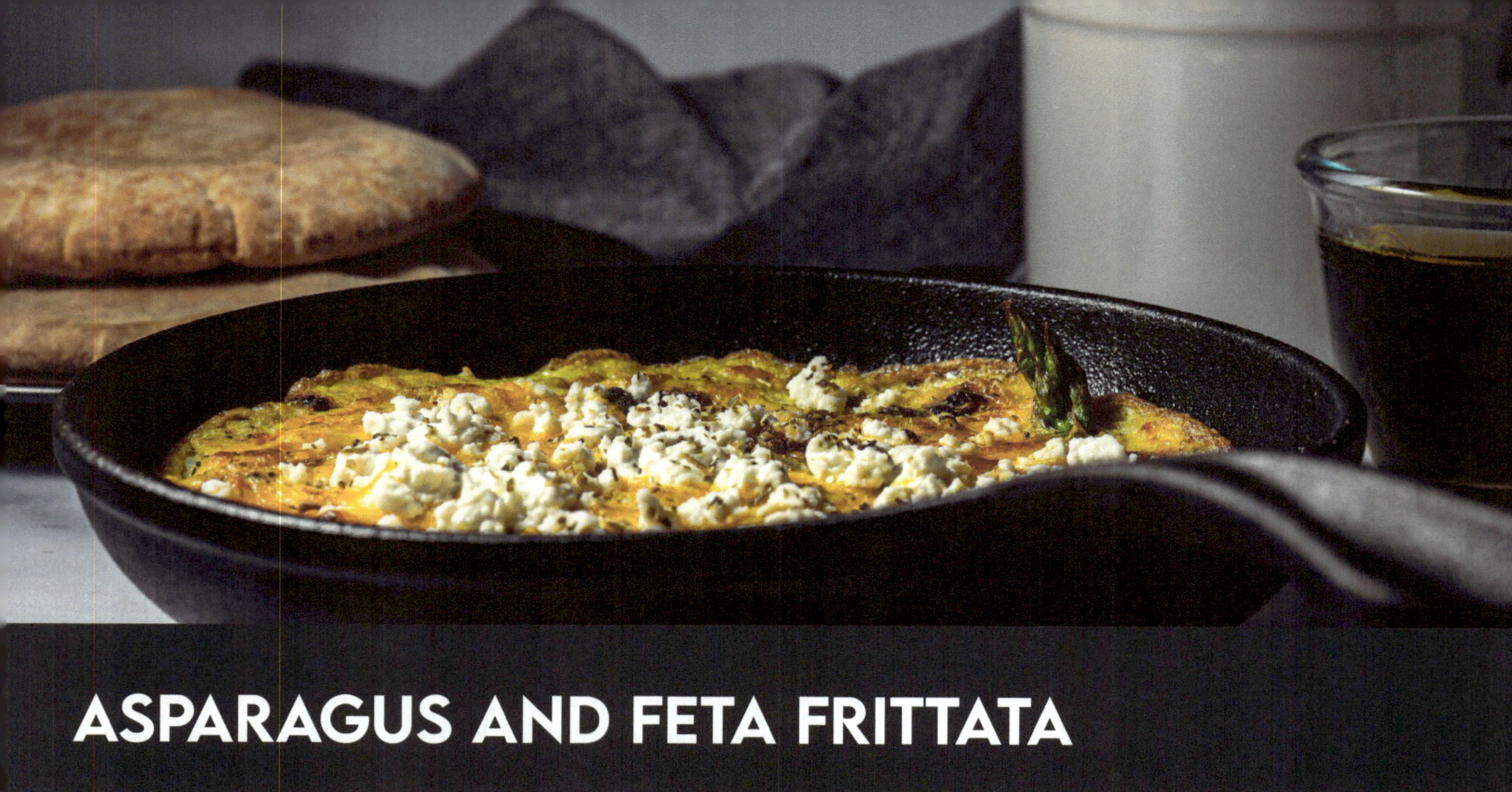

ASPARAGUS AND FETA FRITTATA

Preparation Time	Cooking Time	Servings
15 min	20 min	4

- 8 large eggs
- 1 bunch of asparagus
- 1/2 cup crumbled feta cheese
- 2 tablespoons olive oil
- Salt and pepper to taste

Directions

1. Set your oven's temperature to 375°F (190°C).
2. Beat the eggs in a small mixing bowl and stir in the asparagus pieces and feta cheese. Season with salt and pepper.
3. Warm the olive oil in an oven-safe skillet over moderate heat. Pour in the egg mixture and cook without stirring until the edges start to set, about 5 mins.
4. The frittata is done when the center is no longer jiggly, which usually takes approximately 15 minutes in the oven.

Calories: 270 , Total Fat: 20g , Total Carbohydrates: 5g , Fiber: 2g , Protein: 18g

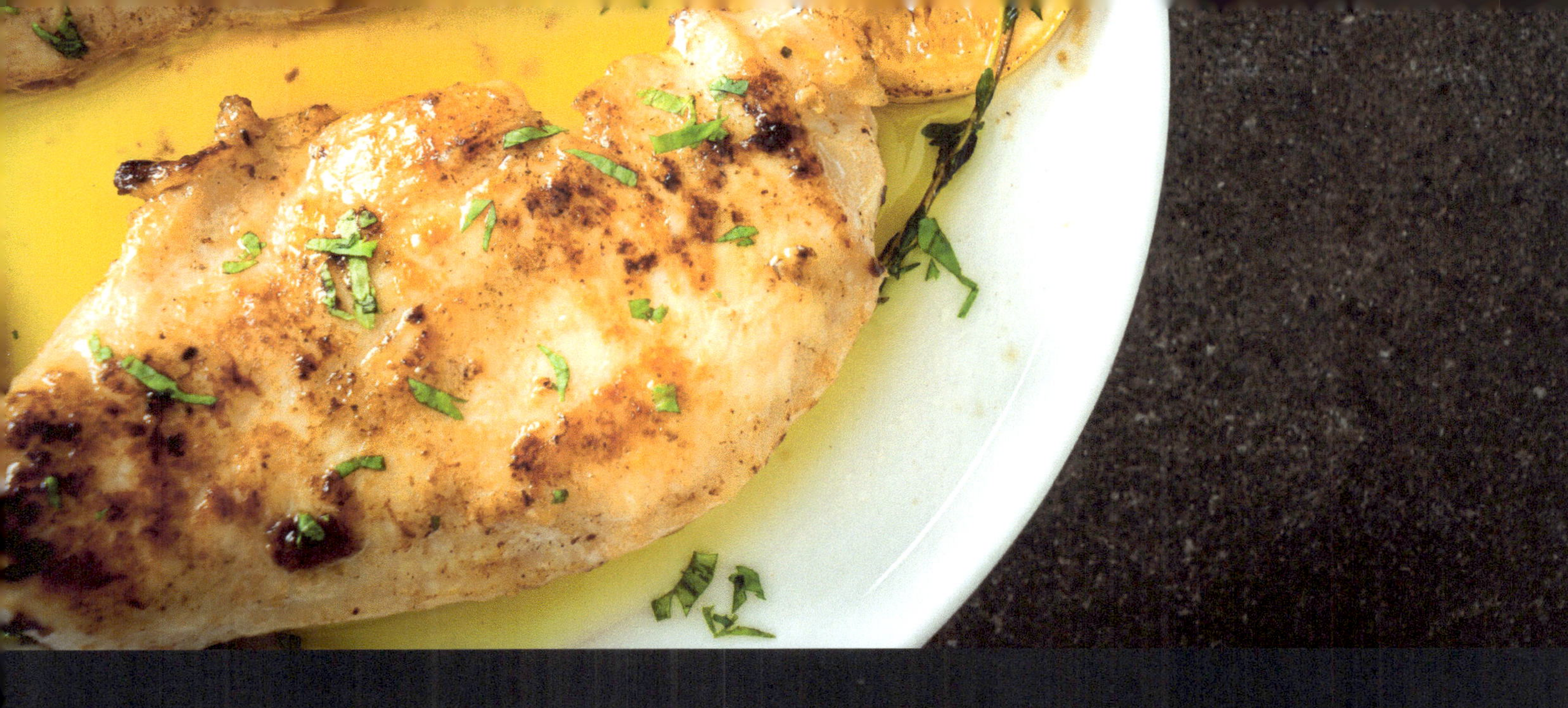

LEMON GARLIC TILAPIA

Preparation Time	Cooking Time	Servings
10 min	20 min	4

- 4 tilapia fillets
- 2 cloves garlic, minced
- Juice and zest of 1 lemon
- 2 tablespoons olive oil
- Salt and pepper to taste

Directions

1. Set your oven's temperature to 375°F (190°C).
2. Arrange the tilapia fillets in a baking dish. Mix the garlic, lemon juice, zest, olive oil, salt & pepper in a small bowl.
3. Pour the lemon garlic mixture over the tilapia fillets. Bake in the preheated oven for 15-20 mins, until the fish flakes with a fork.

Nutrition Information

Calories: 210 , Total Fat: 10g , Total Carbohydrates: 2g , Fiber: 0g , Protein: 28g

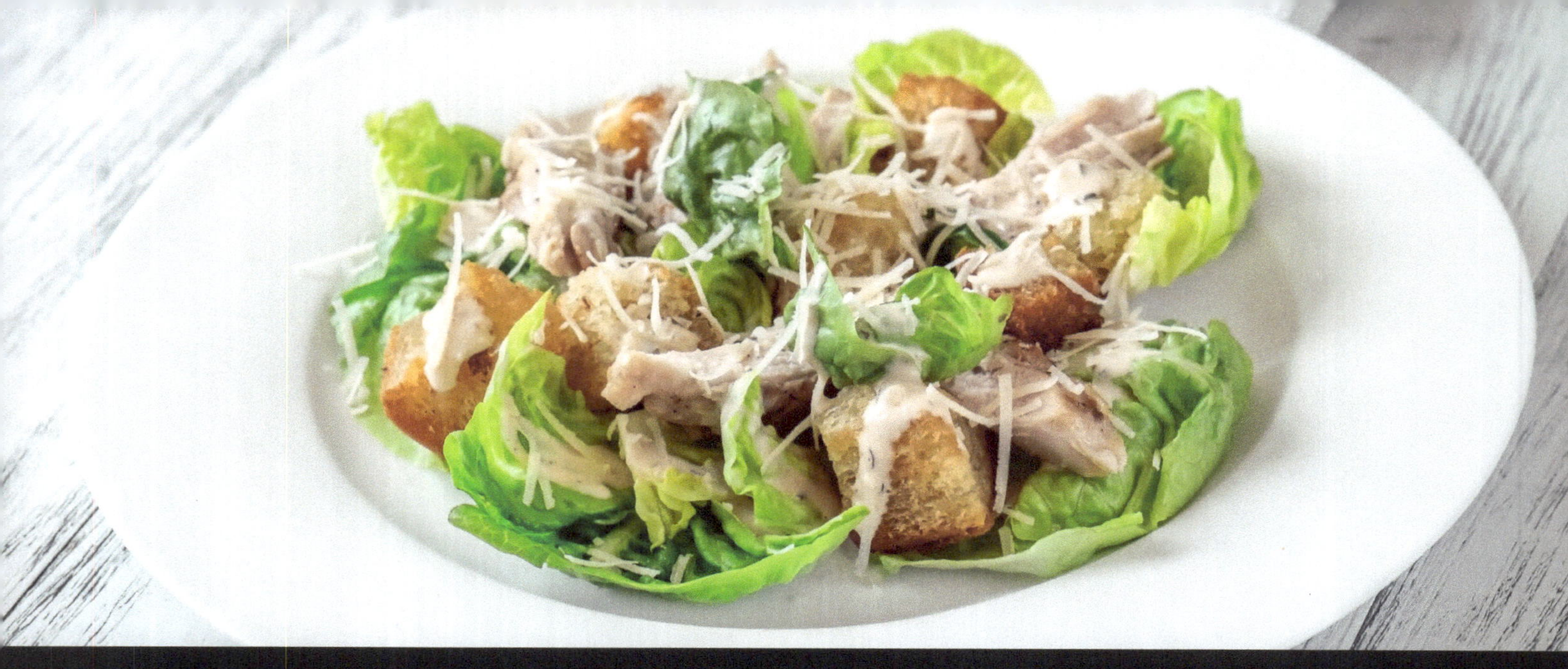

CLASSIC CHICKEN CAESAR

Preparation Time	Cooking Time	Servings
15 min	10 min	4

- 2 boneless, skinless chicken breasts
- 8 cups romaine lettuce, chopped
- 1/2 cup Caesar dressing
- 1/4 cup grated Parmesan cheese
- Salt and pepper to taste

Directions

1. Use salt and pepper to sprinkle the chicken breasts. Grill on medium heat for 5 minutes on each side until cooked through. Let them rest for a few minutes, then slice.
2. Toss the chopped romaine lettuce with the Caesar dressing. Slice the chicken breasts, sprinkle the grated Parmesan on top, and divide it among four dishes.

Nutrition Information

Calories: 330 , Total Fat: 21g , Total Carbohydrates: 8g , Fiber: 3g , Protein: 26g

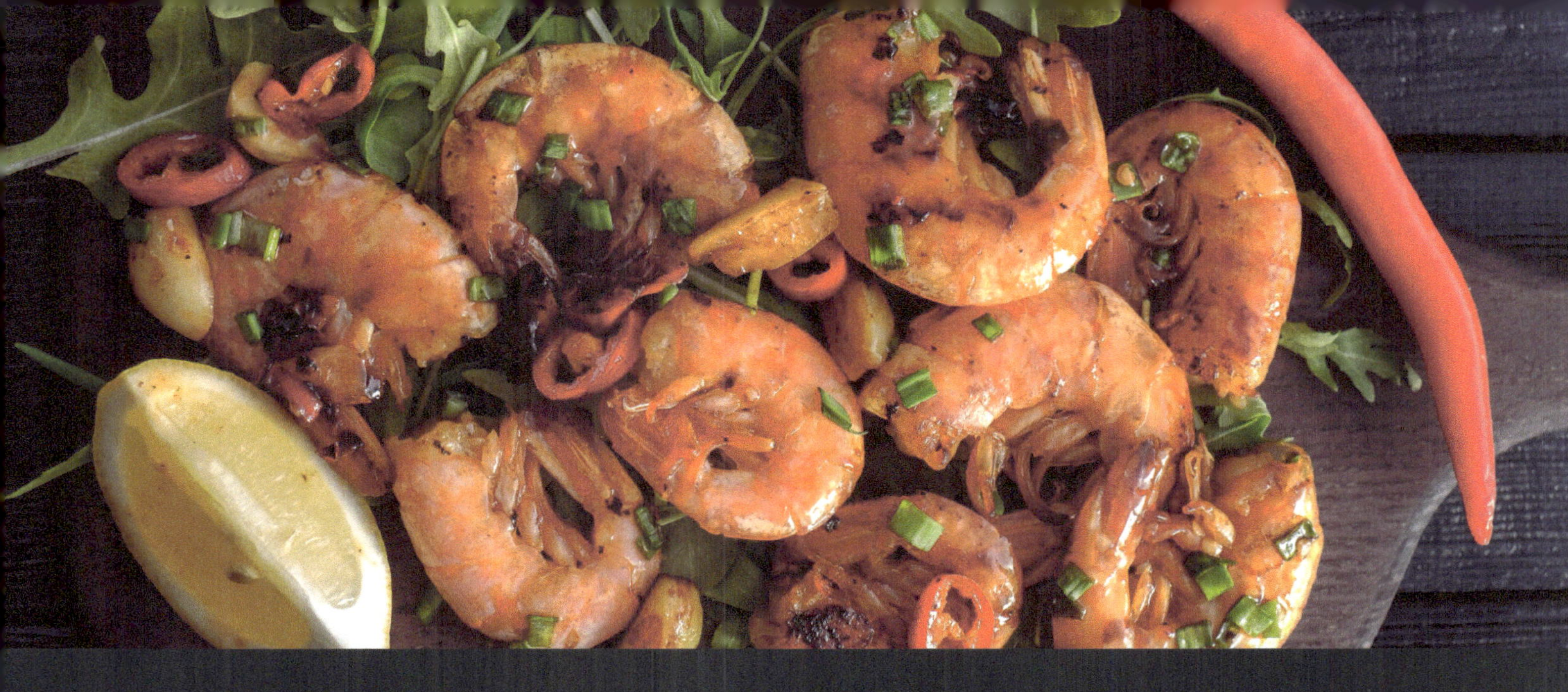

BBQ GRILLED SHRIMP

Preparation Time	Cooking Time	Servings
10 min	10 min	4

- 1 pound large shrimp, peeled and deveined
- 1/2 cup BBQ sauce

Directions

1. Preheat your grill to medium heat. Thread the shrimp onto skewers and brush with BBQ sauce.
2. Grill the shrimp on each side for 2-3 minutes until they're opaque and cooked.

Calories: 170 , Total Fat: 2g , Total Carbohydrates: 10g , Fiber: 0g , Protein: 26g

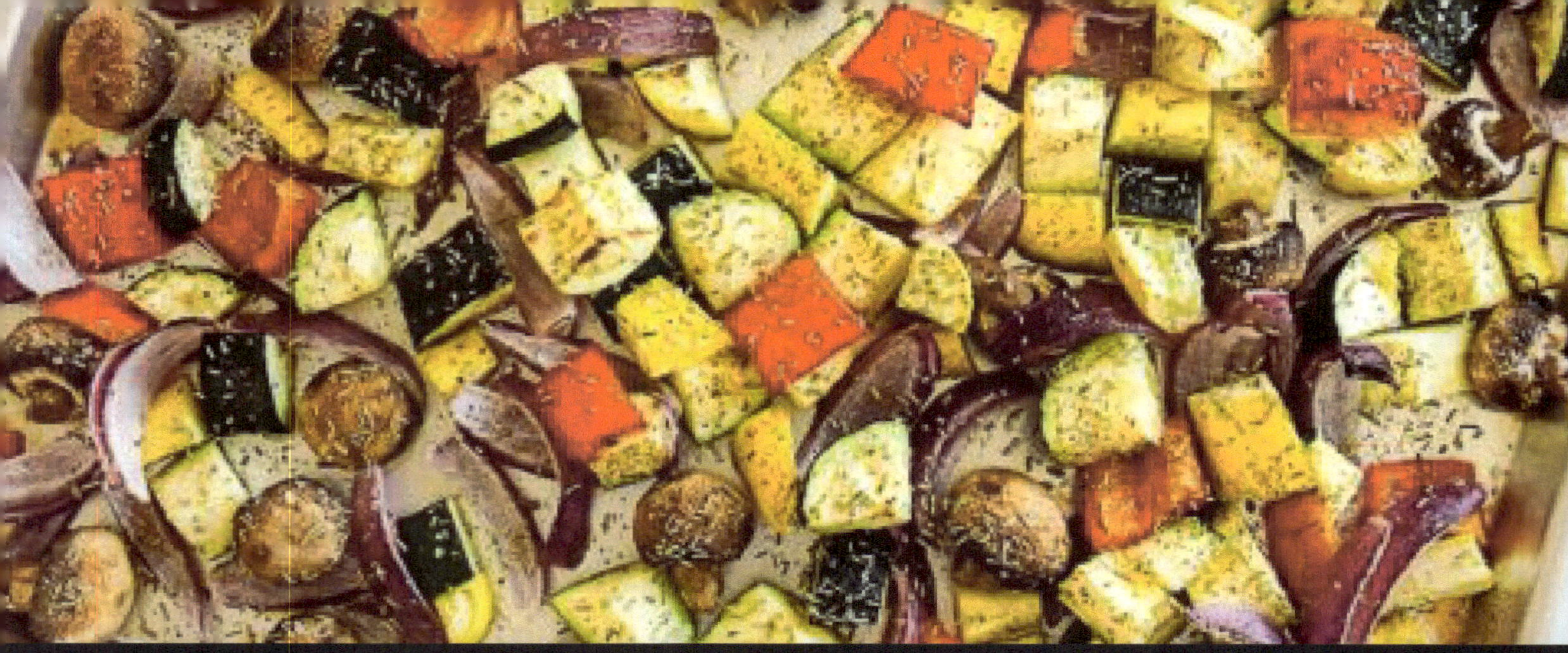

ROASTED VEGGIE MEDLEY

Preparation Time 15 min	Cooking Time 25 min	Servings 4

- 2 bell peppers, cut into 1-inch pieces
- 1 zucchini, cut into 1-inch pieces
- 1 yellow squash, cut into 1-inch pieces
- 1 red onion, cut into 1-inch pieces
- 2 tablespoons olive oil
- Salt and pepper to taste

Directions

1. Set your oven's temperature to 400°F (200°C). Toss to combine vegetables with olive oil, salt & pepper.
2. Spread the vegetables in one layer on a baking tray. Roast in the preheated oven for 25 mins until tender and lightly browned.

Nutrition Information

Calories: 110 , Total Fat: 7g , Total Carbohydrates: 12g , Fiber: 3g , Protein: 2g

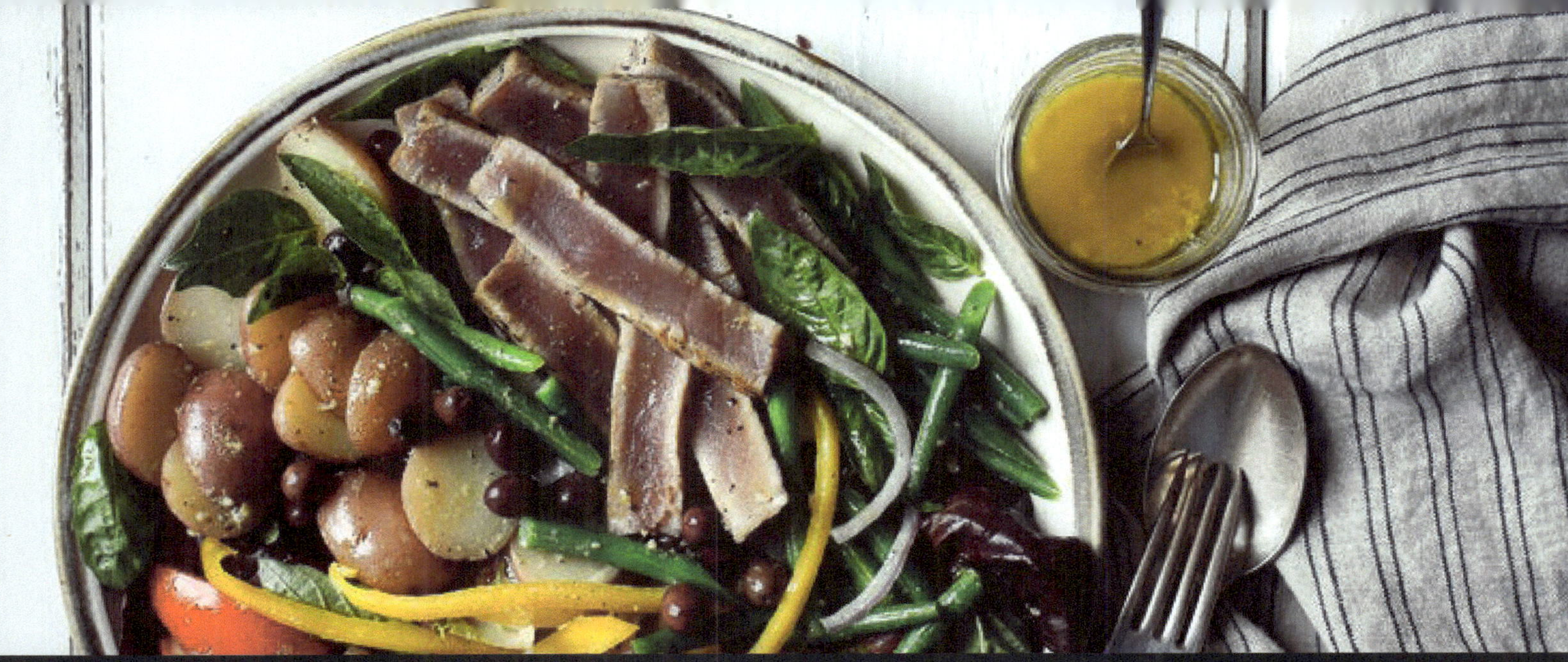

GRILLED TUNA NICOISE

Preparation Time	Cooking Time	Servings
20 min	15 min	4

- 4 tuna steaks
- 4 cups mixed salad greens
- 1 cup cherry tomatoes, halved
- 1/2 cup Kalamata olives
- 1/4 cup red wine vinegar
- 1/2 cup olive oil
- Salt and pepper to taste

Directions

1. Preheat your grill to medium heat. Using salt and pepper, season the tuna steaks.
2. Grill the tuna on each side for 2-3 minutes until cooked to the desired doneness.
3. Divide the salad greens, cherry tomatoes, and olives among four plates. Top each salad with a grilled tuna steak.
4. Mix the red wine vinegar and olive oil in a small bowl with a whisk. Drizzle the dressing over the salads just before serving.

Nutrition Information

Calories: 410, Total Fat: 27g , Total Carbohydrates: 6g , Fiber: 2g
Protein: 35g

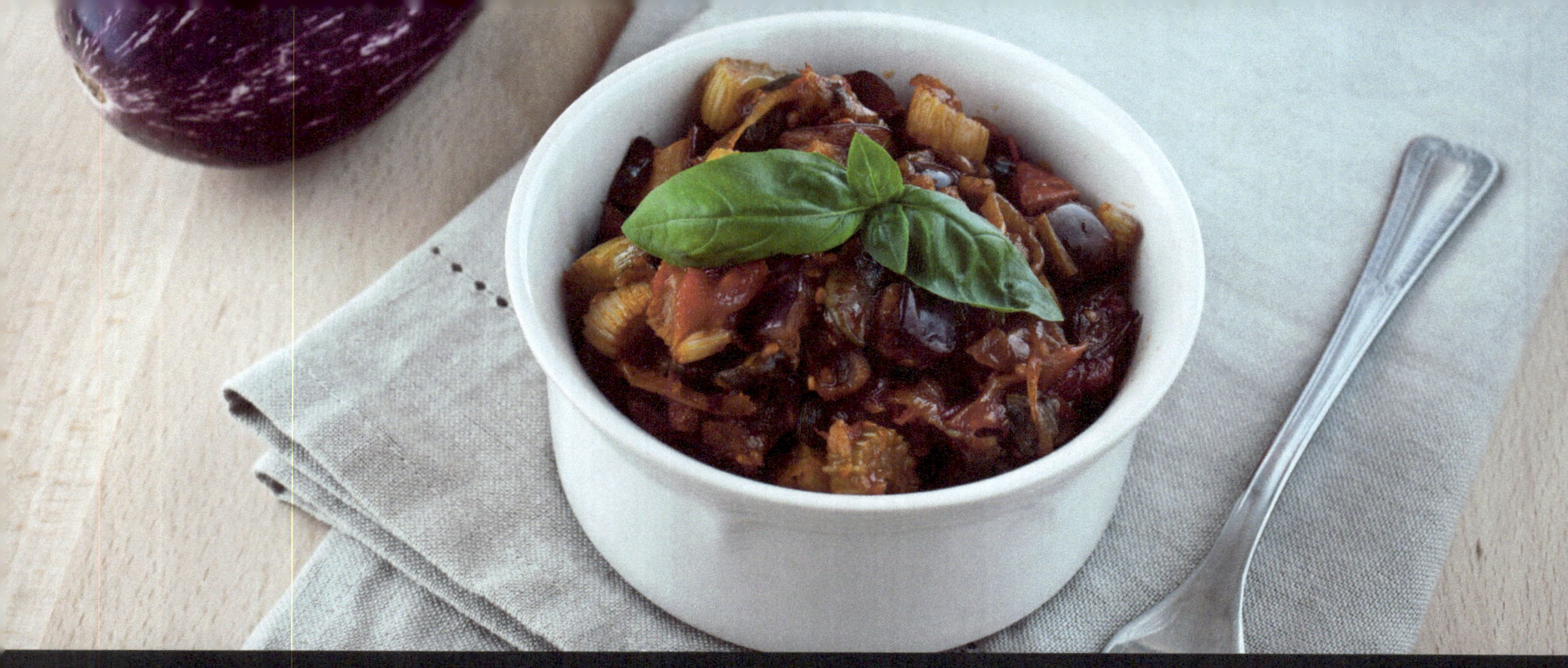

EGGPLANT CAPONATA

Preparation Time	Cooking Time	Servings
15 min	30 min	4

- 1 large eggplant, diced
- 2 tablespoons olive oil
- 1 onion, diced
- 2 cloves garlic, minced
- 1 can diced tomatoes
- 2 tablespoons capers
- 1/4 cup chopped fresh basil
- Salt and pepper to taste

Directions

1. Warm the olive oil in a pan over moderate heat. Add the eggplant and cook until softened about 10 minutes.
2. Add the onion and garlic and continue cooking for 5 minutes.
3. Stir in the diced tomatoes (with juice), capers, and basil. Season with salt and pepper. Simmer for 15 minutes.

Nutrition Information

Calories: 140 , Total Fat: 7g , Total Carbohydrates: 19g , Fiber: 8g , Protein: 3g

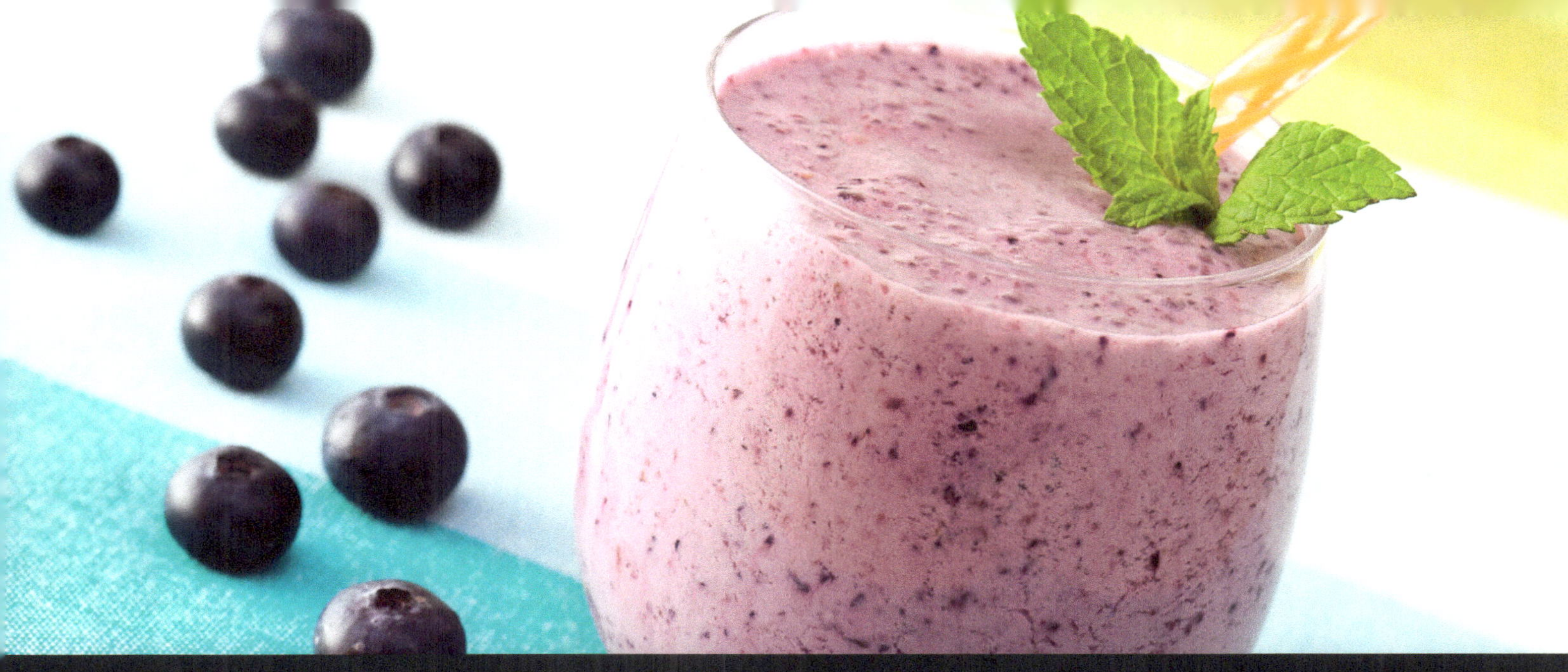

BERRY GREEN SMOOTHIE

Preparation Time	Cooking Time	Servings
5 min	0 min	2

Ingredients

- 1 cup spinach
- 1/2 cup frozen mixed berries
- 1 banana
- 1 cup almond milk

Directions

1. Please put all ingredients in a blender until they are completely smooth.

Nutrition Information

Calories: **120** , Fat: **1g** , Total Carbohydrates: **27g** , Fiber: **5g** , Protein: **3g**

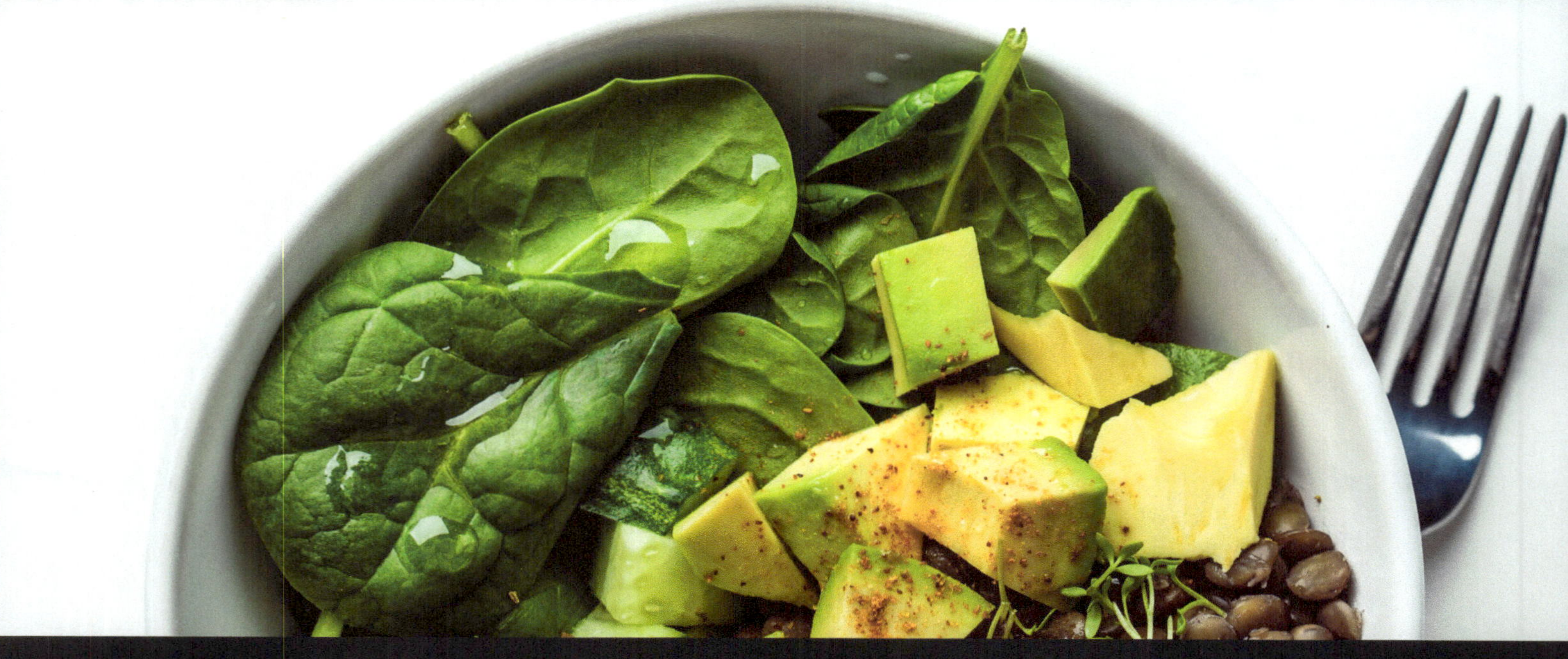

AVOCADO & SPINACH SALAD

<h2>Ingredients</h2>

Preparation Time	Cooking Time	Servings
10 min	0 min	4

- 8 cups spinach
- 2 avocados, sliced
- 1/2 cup sliced almonds
- 1/4 cup olive oil
- 2 tablespoons lemon juice
- Salt and pepper to taste

Directions

1. Divide the spinach, avocados, and sliced almonds among four plates.
2. Whisk together the oil, lime juice, salt & pepper in a small bowl. Drizzle the dressing over the salads.

Nutrition Information

Calories: 320 , Total Fat: 28g , Total Carbohydrates: 16g , Fiber: 10g , Protein: 6g

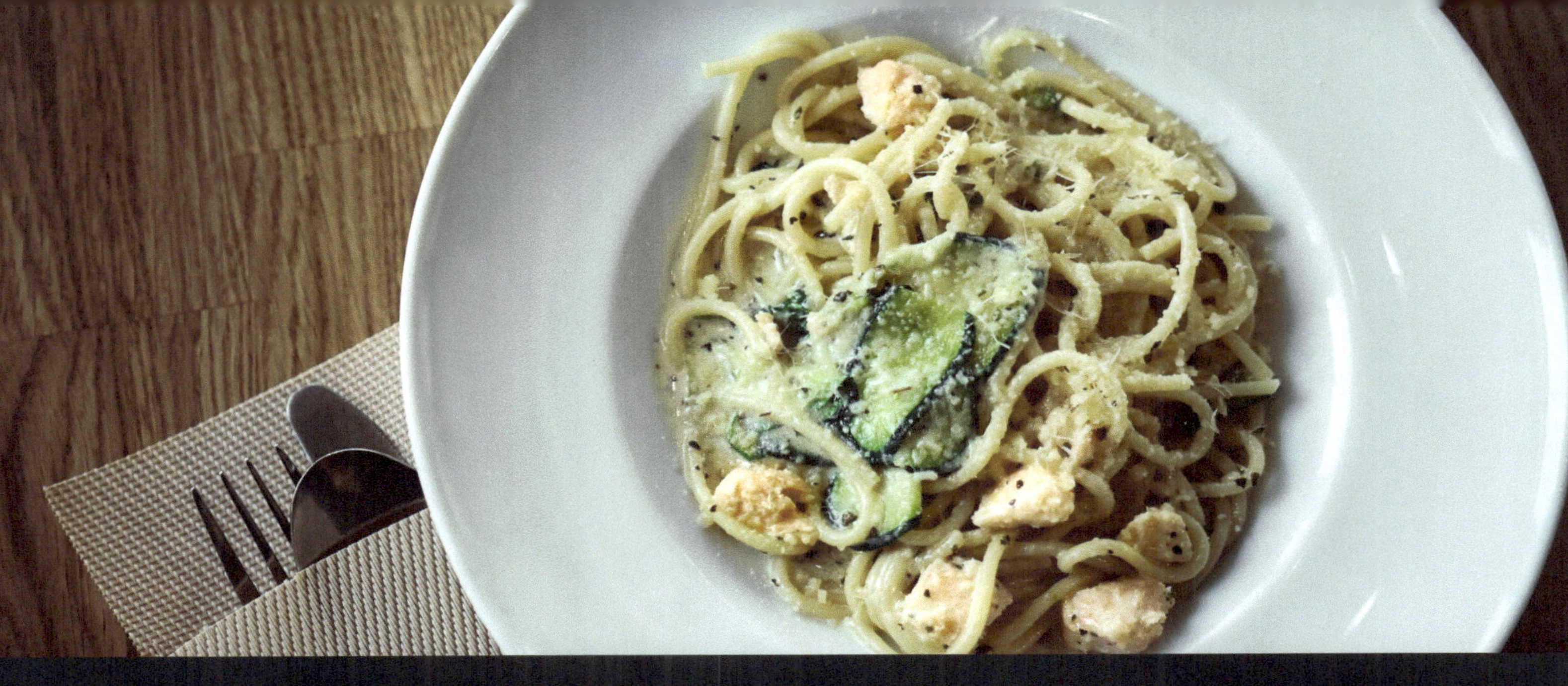

ZUCCHINI NOODLE ALFREDO

Ingredients

Preparation Time	Cooking Time	Servings
10 min	15 min	2

- 2 large zucchinis
- 1 tablespoon olive oil
- 2 cloves garlic, minced
- 1/4 cup low-fat cream cheese
- 1/4 cup grated Parmesan cheese
- Salt and pepper to taste

Directions

1. Spiralize zucchini into noodles.
2. Medium-heat olive oil in a pan. Add the garlic and prepare until fragrant, about 1-2 minutes.
3. Cook zucchini noodles in the pan for 3–4 minutes until soft but crunchy.
4. Melt and mix the cream cheese and Parmesan cheese. Season with salt and pepper.

Nutrition Information

Calories: 210 , Total Fat: 14g , Total Carbohydrates: 14g , Fiber: 4g , Protein: 10g

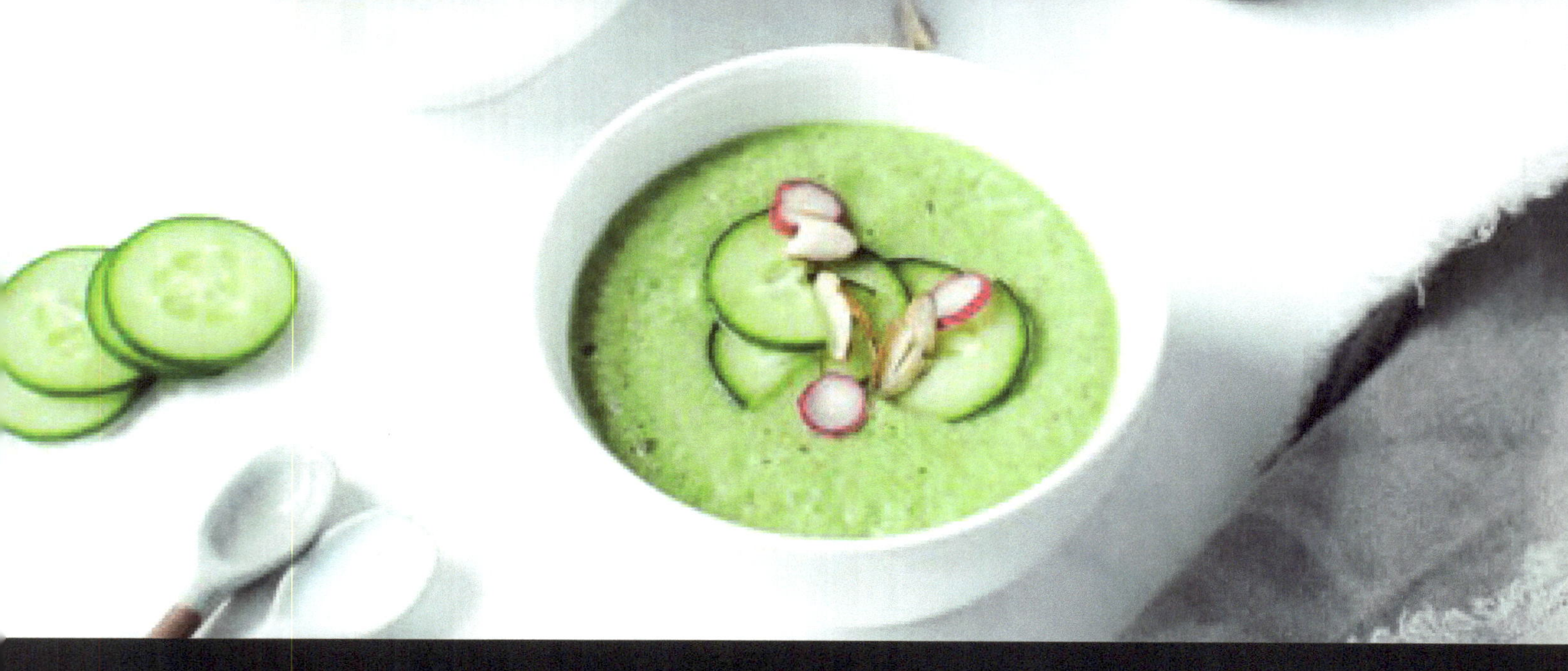

CUCUMBER GAZPACHO

<table>
<tr><td>Preparation Time
15 min</td><td>Cooking Time
0 min</td><td>Servings
4</td></tr>
</table>

Ingredients

- 2 cucumbers, peeled and diced
- 1 green bell pepper, seeded and diced
- 1/2 red onion, diced
- 2 cloves garlic, minced
- 2 tablespoons olive oil
- 2 tablespoons white wine vinegar
- 1 cup low-sodium vegetable broth
- Salt and pepper to taste

Directions

1. Combine the cucumbers, bell pepper, red onion, garlic, olive oil, white wine vinegar, and vegetable broth in a blender. Blend until smooth.
2. Season with salt and pepper to taste. Chill in the freezer for at least 1 hour before serving.

Nutrition Information

Calories: 80 , Total Fat: 6g , Total Carbohydrates: 6g , Fiber: 1g , Protein: 1g

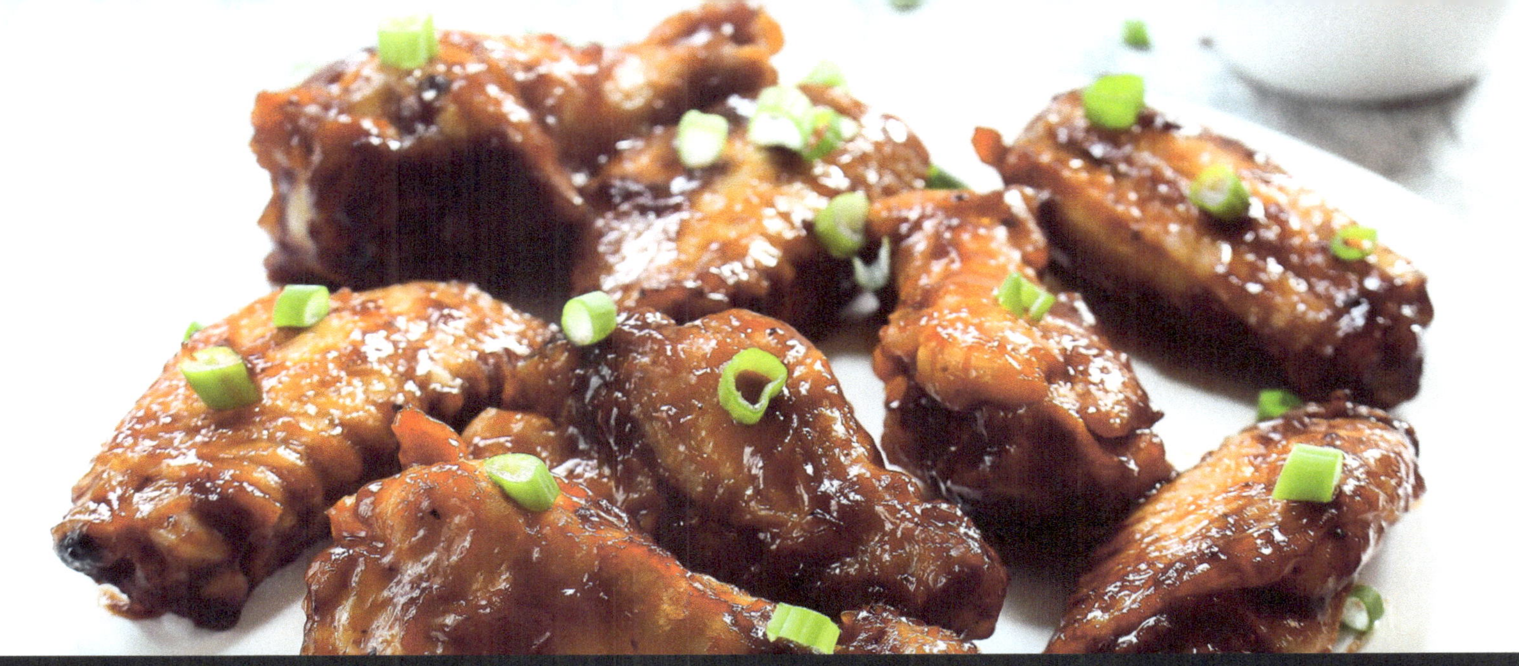

BALSAMIC GLAZED CHICKEN

Ingredients

Preparation Time	Cooking Time	Servings
10 min	20 min	4

- 4 boneless, skinless chicken breasts
- 1/4 cup balsamic vinegar
- 2 tablespoons honey
- 2 cloves garlic, minced
- 1 tablespoon olive oil
- Salt and pepper to taste

Directions

1. Set your grill or grill pan over moderate heat.
2. Season the chicken breasts with salt & pepper.
3. Whisk the balsamic vinegar, honey, garlic, and olive oil in a small bowl.
4. Brush the balsamic glaze onto both sides of the chicken breasts.
5. Grill the chicken for 8-10 mins per side until prepared, and the glaze is caramelized.

Nutrition Information

Calories: 260 , Total Fat: 6g , Total Carbohydrates: 13g , Fiber: 0g , Protein: 38g

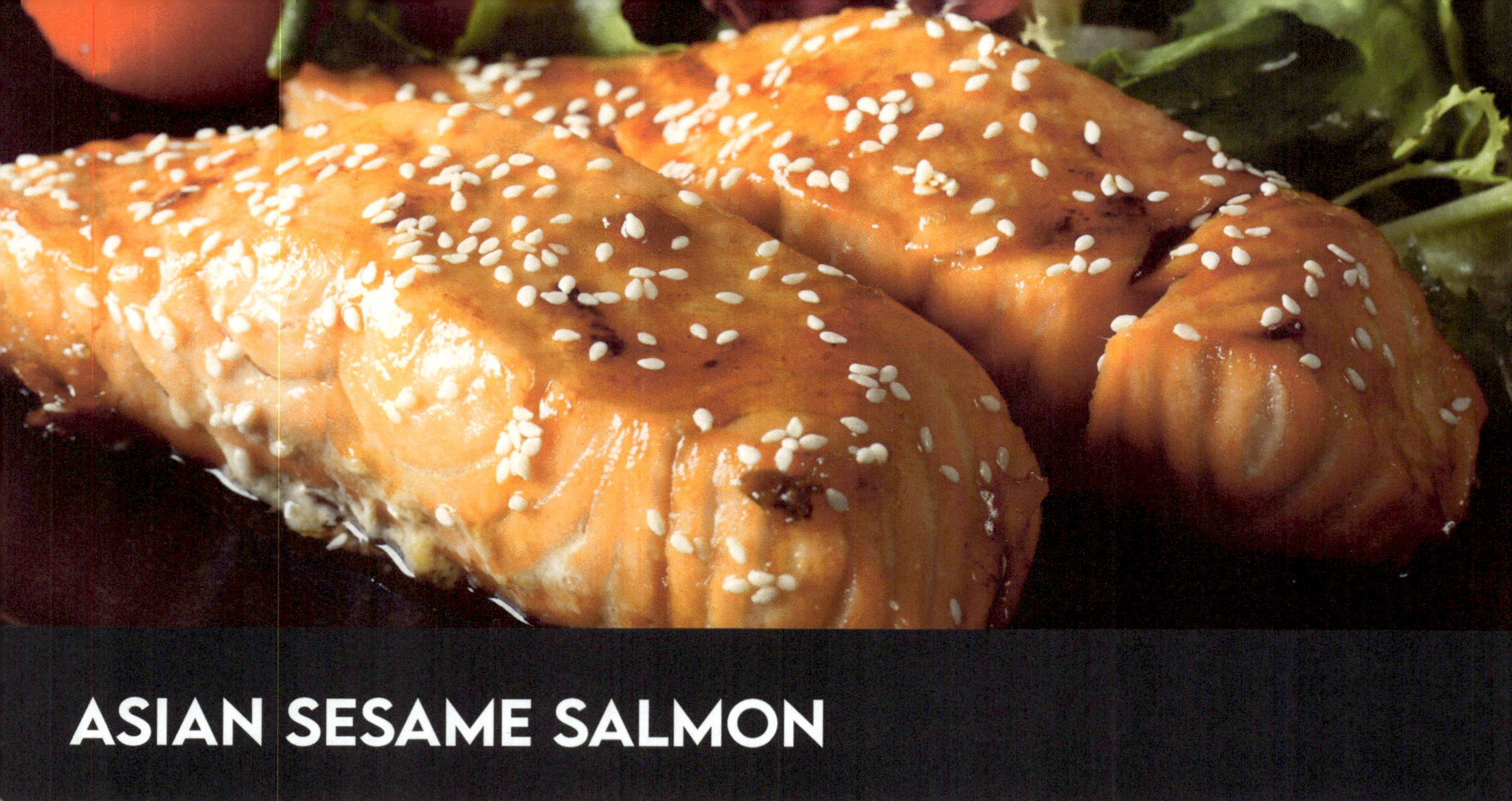

ASIAN SESAME SALMON

Ingredients

Preparation Time	Cooking Time	Servings
10 min	15 min	4

- 4 salmon fillets
- 2 tablespoons low-sodium soy sauce
- 1 tablespoon sesame oil
- 1 tablespoon honey
- 2 cloves garlic, minced
- 1 teaspoon grated fresh ginger
- 1 tablespoon sesame seeds
- Salt and pepper to taste

Directions

1. Adjust your oven to 375°F (190°C).
2. Whisk the soy sauce, sesame oil, honey, garlic, ginger, sesame seeds, salt, and pepper in a small bowl.
3. Set the salmon fillets on a baking tray lined with parchment paper. Pour the sauce over the salmon.
4. Bake in the heated oven for 12-15 mins or until the salmon is prepared to your desired doneness.

Nutrition Information

Calories: 300 , Total Fat: 18g , Total Carbohydrates: 5g , Fiber: 0g , Protein: 30g

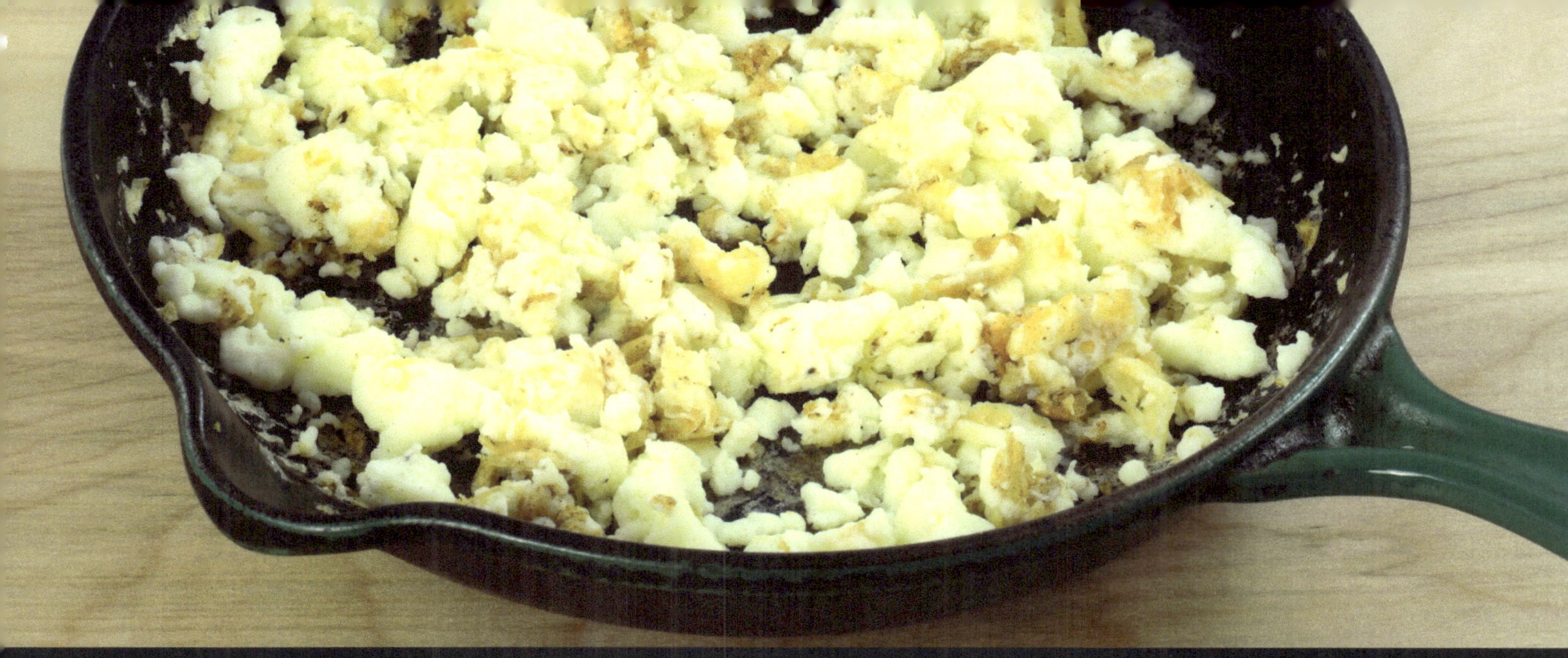

EGG WHITE SCRAMBLE

Preparation Time	Cooking Time	Servings
5 min	10 min	2

- 6 egg whites
- 1 cup spinach
- 1/4 cup diced bell peppers
- 1/4 cup diced onions
- 2 tablespoons grated Parmesan cheese
- Salt and pepper to taste
- Cooking spray

Directions

1. Spray a non-stick skillet with spray (cooking) and place it over medium heat.
2. Put the onions and bell peppers in the pan and prepare until softened about 2-3 mins.
3. Add the egg whites and spinach to the skillet. Cook, stirring occasionally, until the egg whites are set, about 5 minutes.
4. Season with salt & pepper, and sprinkle with grated Parmesan cheese.

Nutrition Information

Calories: 90 , Total Fat: 2g , Total Carbohydrates: 4g , Fiber: 1g , Protein: 16g

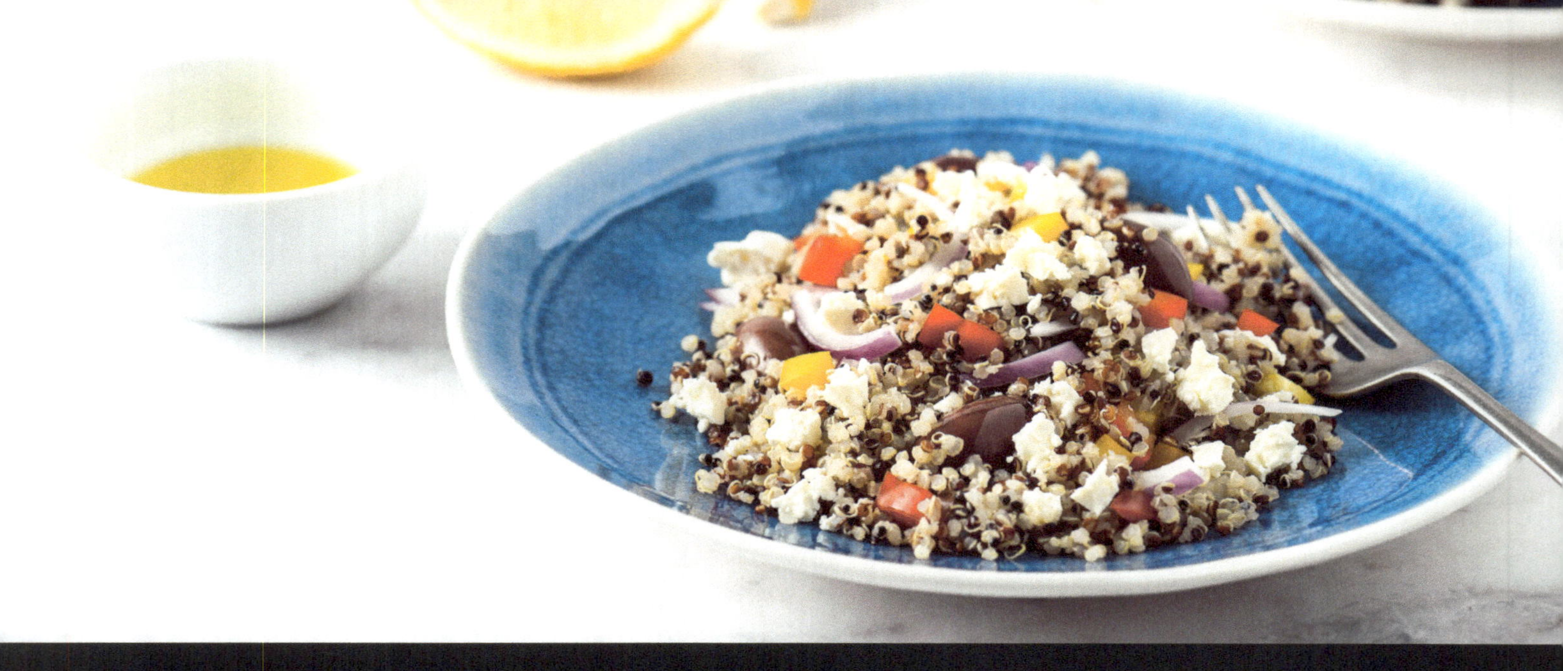

MEDITERRANEAN QUINOA SALAD

Ingredients

Preparation Time	Cooking Time	Servings
15 min	15 min	4

- 1 cup cooked quinoa
- 1 cup diced cucumbers
- 1 cup cherry tomatoes, halved
- 1/4 cup sliced Kalamata olives
- 1/4 cup crumbled feta cheese
- 2 tablespoons chopped fresh parsley
- 2 tablespoons lemon juice
- 2 tablespoons extra-virgin olive oil
- Salt and pepper to taste

Directions

1. Combine the cooked quinoa, cucumbers, cherry tomatoes, olives, feta cheese, and parsley in a large bowl.
2. Mix the lime juice, olive oil, salt, and pepper in a small bowl. Pour the dressing on the quinoa salad and toss to combine.

Nutrition Information

Calories: 220, Total Fat: 12g , Total Carbohydrates: 22g , Fiber: 4g
Protein: 7g

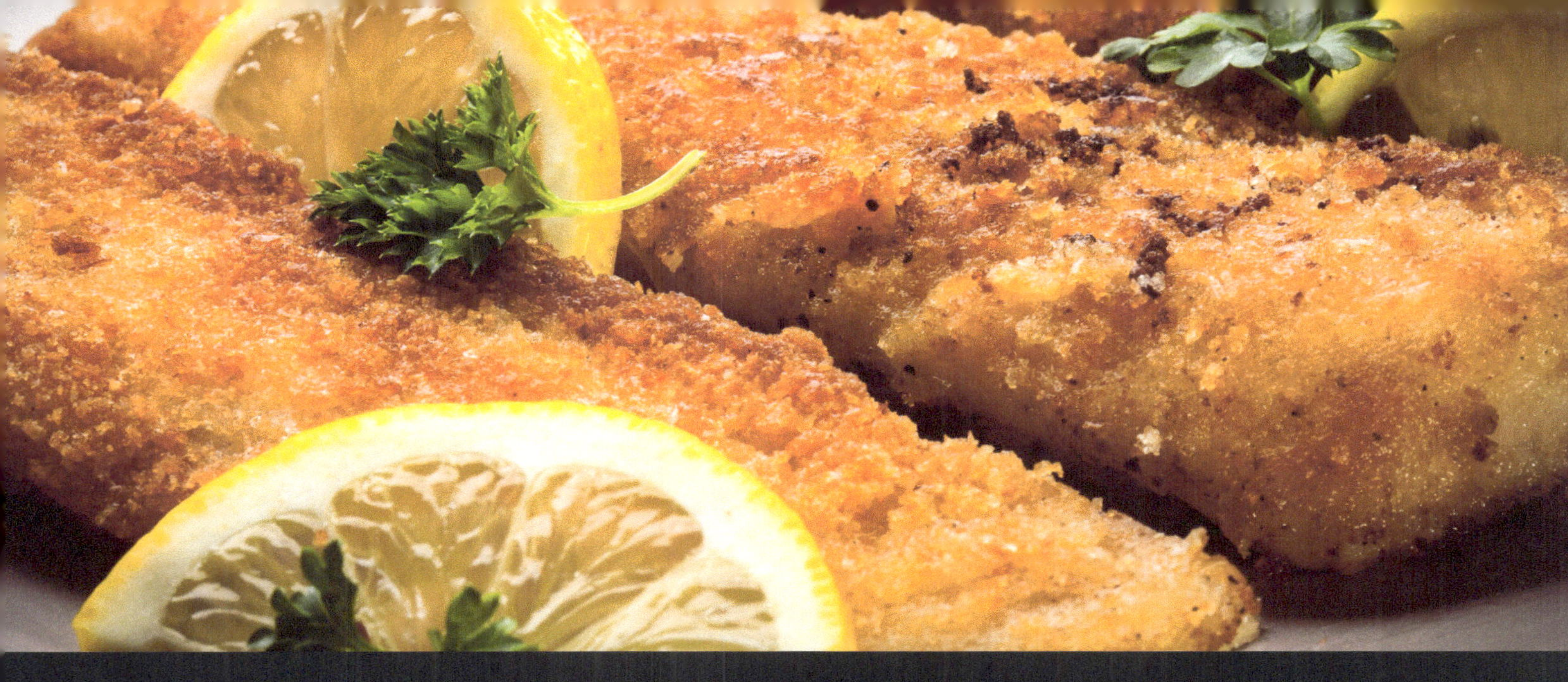

CAJUN GRILLED COD

<table>
<tr><th>Preparation Time
10 min</th><th>Cooking Time
10 min</th><th>Servings
4</th></tr>
</table>

Ingredients

- 4 cod fillets
- 2 tablespoons Cajun seasoning
- 1 tablespoon olive oil
- Salt and pepper to taste

Directions

1. Preheat your grill to medium heat.
2. Rub the cod fillets with Cajun seasoning, olive oil, salt, and pepper.
3. Grill the cod on each side for 4-5 mins until the fish flakes easily with a fork.

Nutrition Information

Calories: 150, Total Fat: 4g , Total Carbohydrates: 2g , Fiber: 1g
Protein: 26g

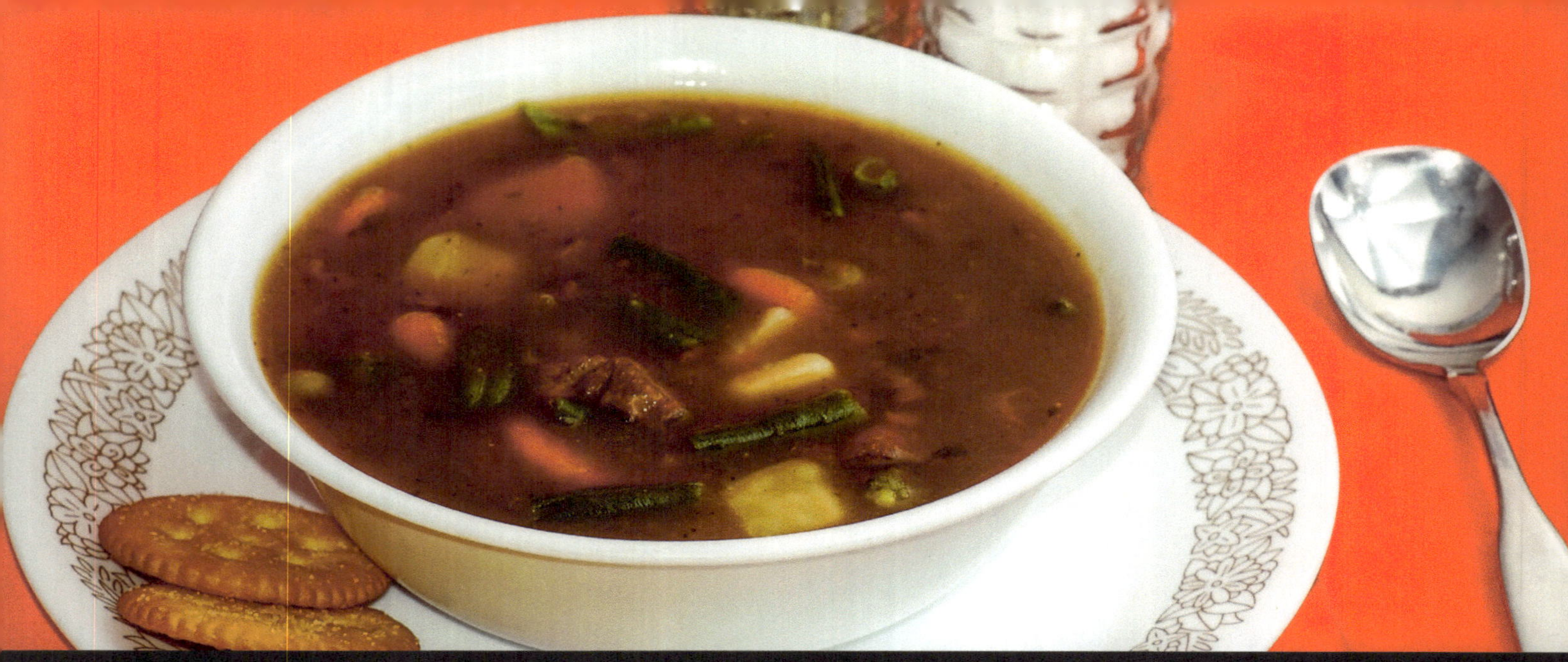

HEARTY VEGETABLE STEW

Preparation Time	Cooking Time	Servings
15 min	30 min	6

- 1 tablespoon olive oil
- 1 onion, diced
- 2 carrots, peeled and sliced
- 2 celery stalks, sliced
- 2 cloves garlic, minced
- 4 cups vegetable broth
- 1 can diced tomatoes
- 1 cup diced potatoes
- 1 cup green beans, trimmed and halved
- 1 cup corn kernels
- 1 teaspoon dried thyme
- Salt and pepper to taste

Directions

1. Warm the olive oil in a large pot over moderate heat. Add the onion, carrots, celery, and garlic. Prepare until the vegetables are soft, about 5 mins.
2. Add the vegetable broth, diced tomatoes, potatoes, green beans, corn kernels, dried thyme, salt, & pepper. Take to a boil, then reduce heat and simmer for 20 mins or until the vegetables are cooked.

Nutrition Information

Calories: 180 , Total Fat: 3g , Total Carbohydrates: 36g , Fiber: 8g , Protein: 5g

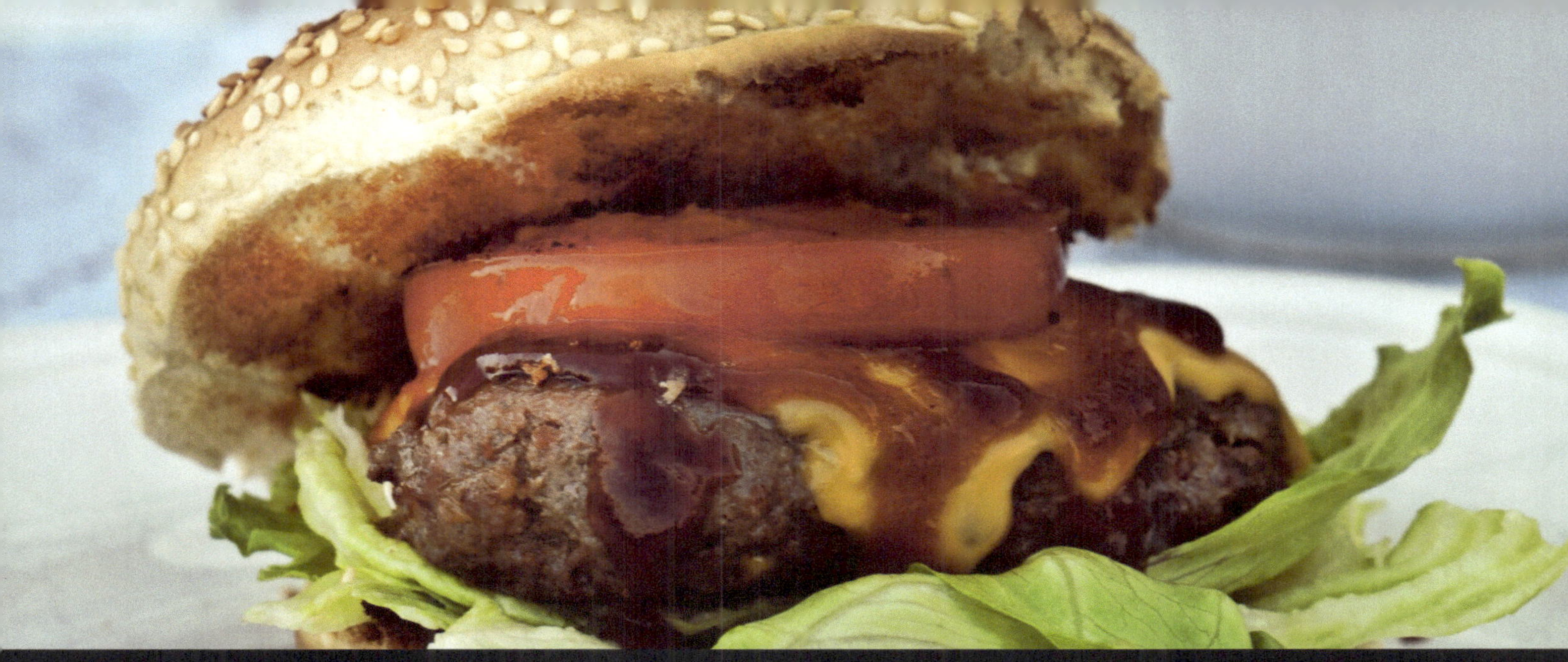

GRILLED TURKEY BURGER

Preparation Time 10 min	Cooking Time 12 min	Servings 4

- 1 pound ground turkey
- 1/4 cup breadcrumbs
- 1/4 cup finely chopped onion
- 1/4 cup chopped fresh parsley
- 1 clove garlic, minced
- 1 teaspoon Worcestershire sauce
- Salt and pepper to taste
- 4 whole wheat burger buns
- Lettuce, tomato, and other desired toppings

Directions

1. Preheat your grill to medium heat.
2. Combine the ground turkey, breadcrumbs, onion, parsley, garlic, Worcestershire sauce, salt & pepper in a bowl. Mix well.
3. Shape the mixture into four patties. Grill the turkey burgers for about 6 minutes on each side or until cooked through.
4. Serve the turkey burgers over whole wheat buns with your preferred toppings.

Nutrition Information

Calories: 250 , Total Fat: 6g , Total Carbohydrates: 24g , Fiber: 4g , Protein: 26g

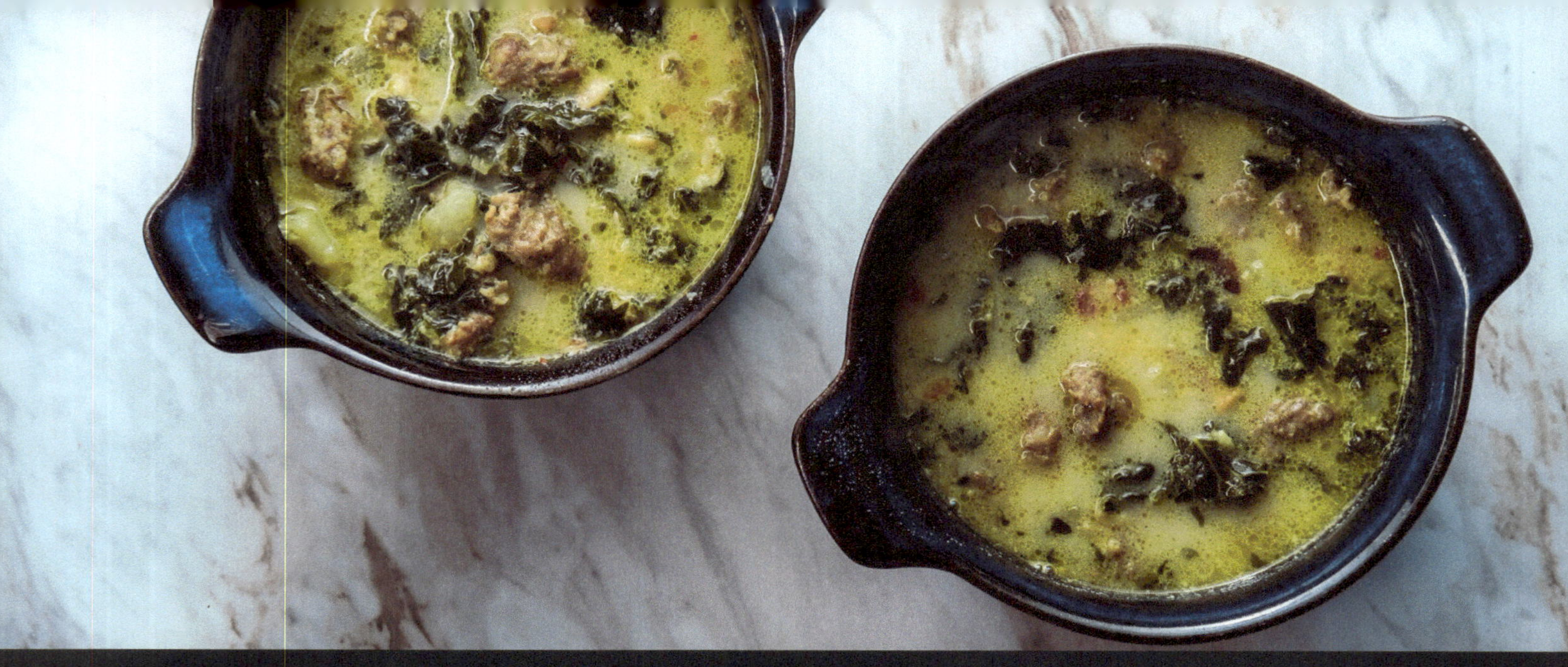

TUSCAN KALE SOUP

Preparation Time	Cooking Time	Servings
15 min	30 min	6

- 1 tablespoon olive oil
- 1 onion, diced
- 2 cloves garlic, minced
- 2 carrots, peeled and sliced
- 2 celery stalks, sliced
- 4 cups vegetable broth
- 1 can diced tomatoes
- 2 cups chopped kale
- 1 can cannellini beans, drained and rinsed
- 1 teaspoon dried Italian seasoning
- Salt and pepper to taste

Directions

1. Warm the olive oil in a large pot over moderate heat. Add the onion, garlic, carrots, and celery. Cook until the vegetables gets softened, about 5 mins.
2. Add the vegetable broth, diced tomatoes, kale, cannellini beans, dried Italian seasoning, salt, and pepper. Take to a boil, then reduce heat and simmer for 20 minutes.

Nutrition Information

Calories: 180 , Total Fat: 3g , Total Carbohydrates: 31g , Fiber: 9g , Protein: 9g

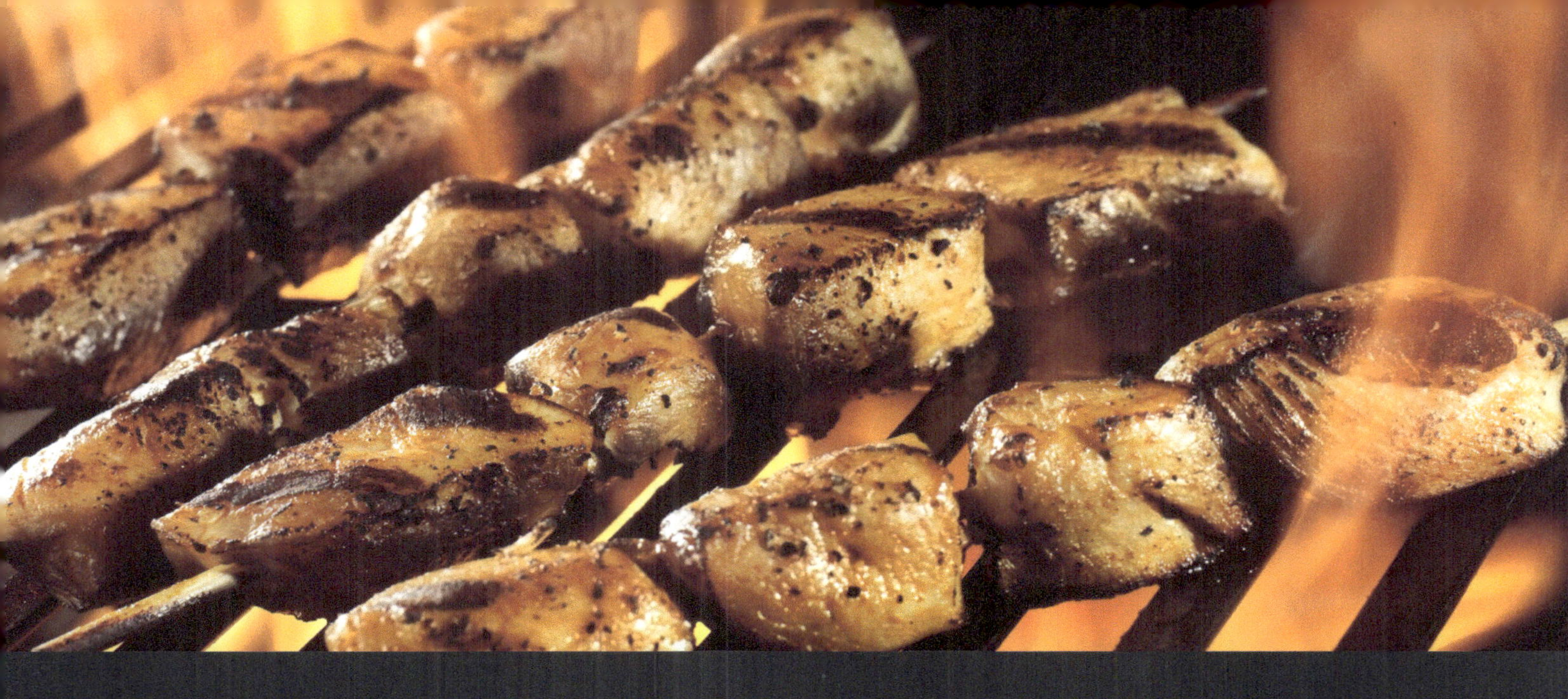

BBQ CHICKEN KEBABS

Preparation Time	Cooking Time	Servings
20 min	15 min	4

- 1 pound boneless, skinless breasts of chicken cut into chunks
- 1/2 cup BBQ sauce
- 1 tablespoon olive oil
- 1 teaspoon smoked paprika
- 1/2 teaspoon garlic powder
- Salt and pepper to taste
- 1 red onion, cut into chunks
- 1 red bell pepper, cut into chunks
- 1 green bell pepper, cut into chunks

Directions

1. Mix the chicken pieces, BBQ sauce, olive oil, smoked paprika, garlic powder, salt & pepper in a bowl. Mix well to coat the chicken.
2. Thread the marinated chicken, red onion, and bell peppers onto skewers.
3. Preheat your grill to medium heat. Grill the chicken kebabs for 6-8 mins on each side or the chicken is cooked and the vegetables are tender.

Nutrition Information

Calories: 250 , Total Fat: 6g , Total Carbohydrates: 19g , Fiber: 2g , Protein: 30g

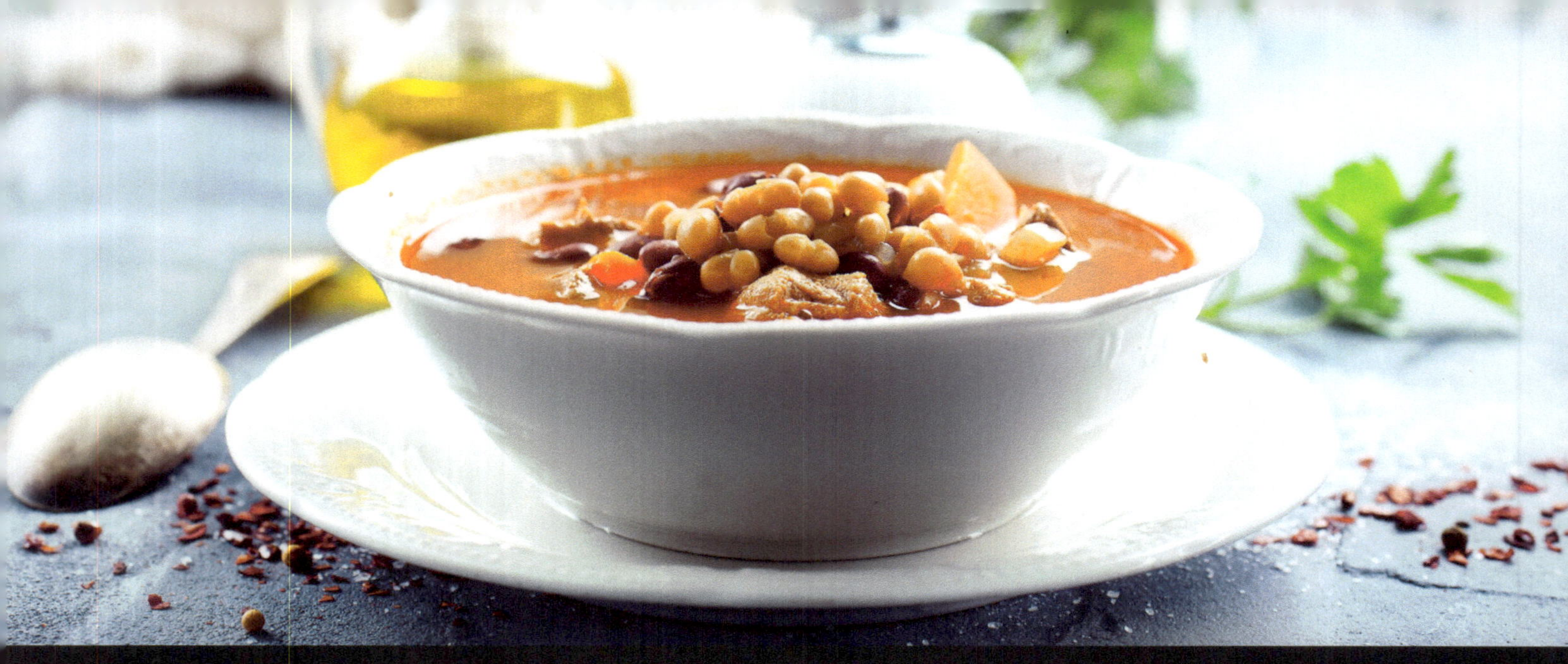

SPICY BLACK BEAN SOUP

<table>
<tr><th>Preparation Time
10 min</th><th>Cooking Time
25 min</th><th>Servings
4</th></tr>
</table>

Ingredients

- 2 tablespoons olive oil
- 1 onion, diced
- 2 cloves garlic, minced
- 1 red bell pepper, diced
- 2 teaspoons chili powder
- 1 teaspoon cumin
- 1/2 teaspoon smoked paprika
- 2 cans black beans, drained and rinsed
- 4 cups vegetable broth
- Juice of 1 lime
- Salt and pepper to taste

Directions

1. Medium-heat olive oil in a saucepan. Add the chopped onion, garlic, and red bell pepper. Prepare until the vegetables are tender, about 5 mins.
2. Combine chili powder, cumin, and smoked paprika. Cook another minute.
3. Add black beans and vegetable broth to the pot. Boil, then simmer for 15 minutes.
4. Use an immersion blender processer to mix the soup partially.
5. Add lime juice and salt & pepper to taste.

Nutrition Information

Calories: **230**, Total Fat: **7g** , Total Carbohydrates: **34g** , Fiber: **11g**
Protein: **9g**

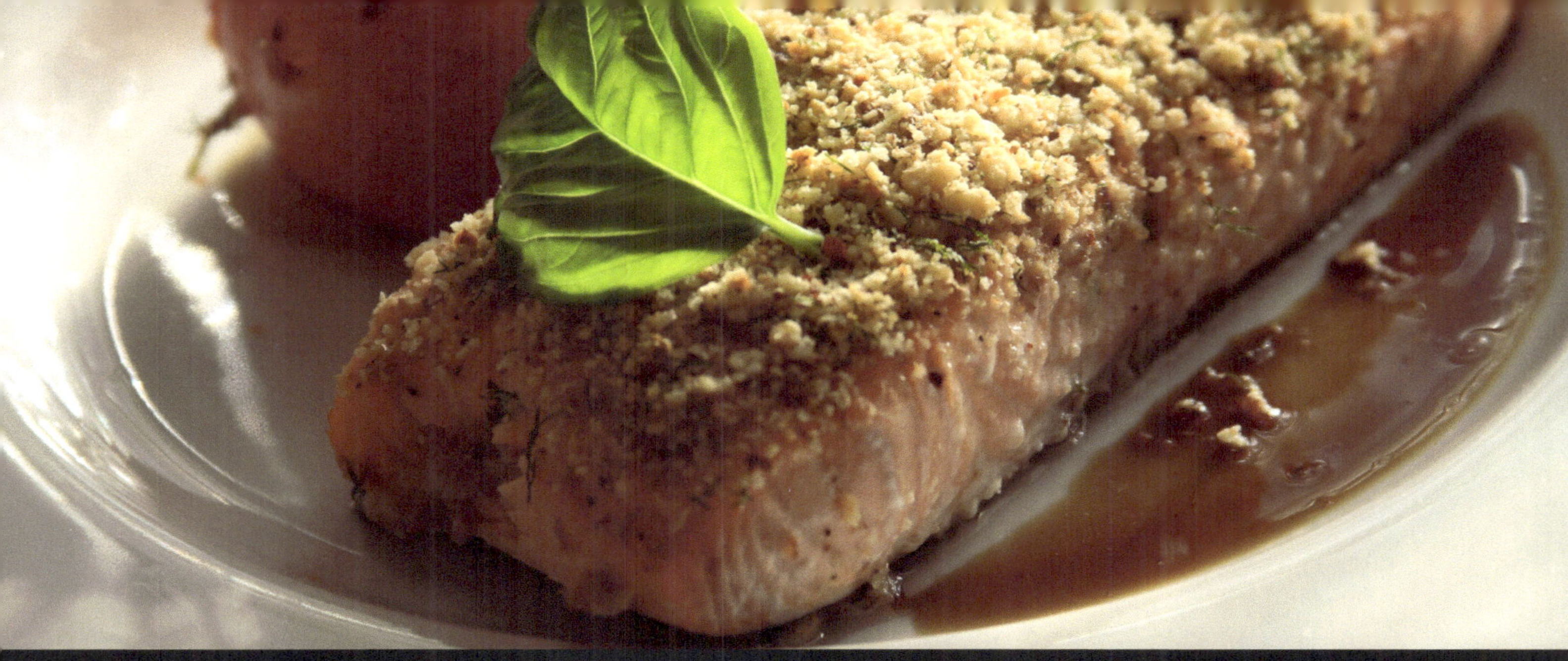

MANGO GRILLED FISH TACOS

<table>
<tr><td>**Preparation Time**
15 min</td><td>**Cooking Time**
10 min</td><td>**Servings**
4</td></tr>
</table>

Ingredients

- 1 lb. of white fish fillets (such as tilapia or cod)
- 2 tablespoons olive oil
- 1 tablespoon lime juice
- 1 teaspoon chili powder
- 1/2 teaspoon cumin
- Salt and pepper to taste
- 8 small corn tortillas
- 1 cup shredded cabbage
- 1 ripe mango, diced
- 1/4 cup chopped fresh cilantro
- Lime wedges for serving

Directions

1. Adjust your grill or grill pan to medium heat.
2. Mix the olive oil, lime juice, chili powder, cumin, salt, & pepper in a small bowl. Brush the fish fillets with the mixture.
3. Grill the fish for 3-4 mins on each side or until prepared through and flaky.
4. On the grill, warm the maize tortillas for 30 seconds per side.
5. Flake the grilled fish into pieces and divide among the warmed tortillas.
6. Top each taco with shredded cabbage, diced mango, and chopped cilantro.
7. Serve the tacos with lemon wedges for squeezing over the top.

Nutrition Information

Calories: 280 , Total Fat: 10g , Total Carbohydrates: 28g , Fiber: 5g , Protein: 20g

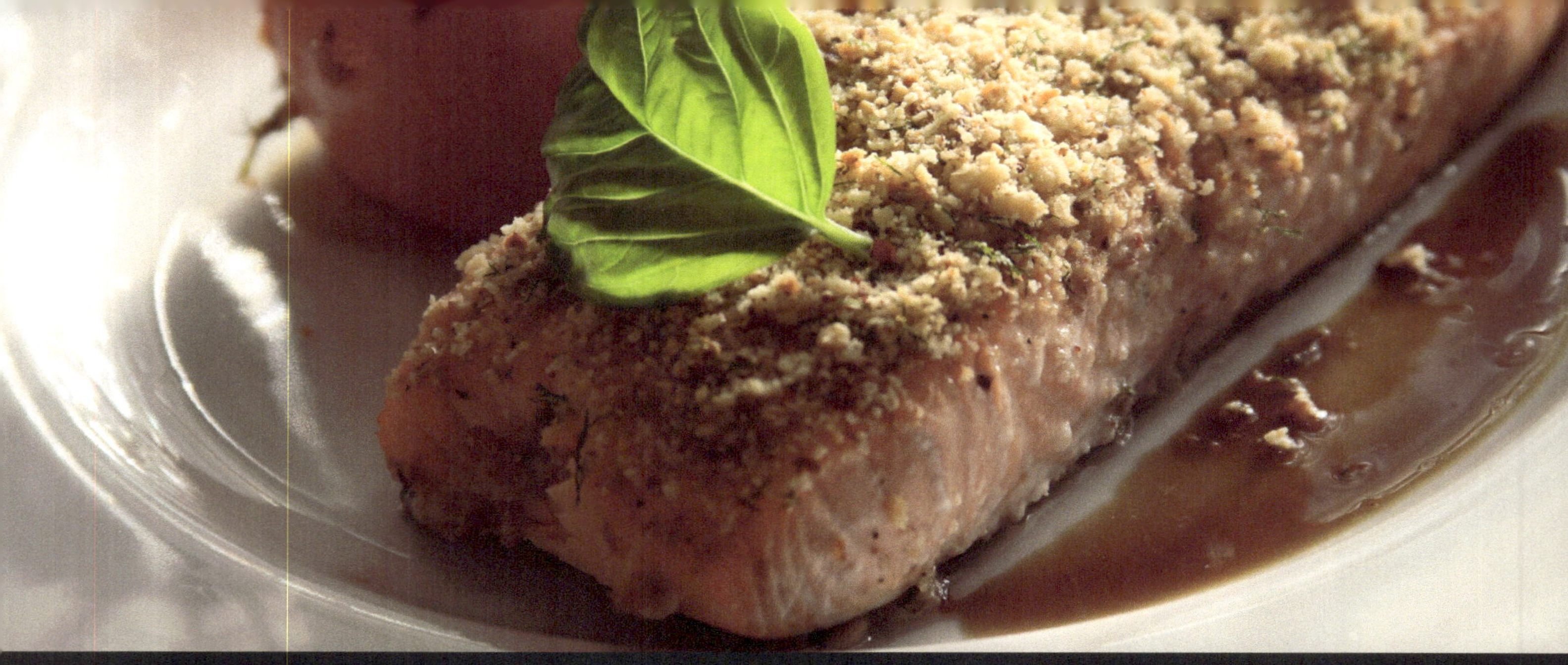

ALMOND CRUSTED TILAPIA

Ingredients

Preparation Time	Cooking Time	Servings
10 min	12 min	4

- 4 tilapia fillets
- 1/4 cup almond flour
- 1/4 cup finely chopped almonds
- 1 teaspoon paprika
- 1/2 teaspoon garlic powder
- Salt and pepper to taste
- 2 tablespoons olive oil
- Lemon wedges for serving

Directions

1. Set your oven's temperature to 400°F (200°C).
2. Combine the almond flour, chopped almonds, paprika, garlic powder, salt, and pepper in a shallow bowl.
3. Use a paper towel to dry the tilapia fillets. Dip each fillet into the almond mixture, pressing gently to coat both sides.
4. Warm the olive oil in an oven-safe skillet over moderate heat. Add the tilapia fillets and cook for 2 minutes on each side to brown.
5. Move the skillet to the heated oven and bake for an additional 8-10 mins, until the fish is cooked and the almond crust is golden.
6. Serve the almond-crusted tilapia with lemon wedges on the side.

Nutrition Information

Calories: 220 , Total Fat: 13g , Total Carbohydrates: 2g , Fiber: 1g , Protein: 24g

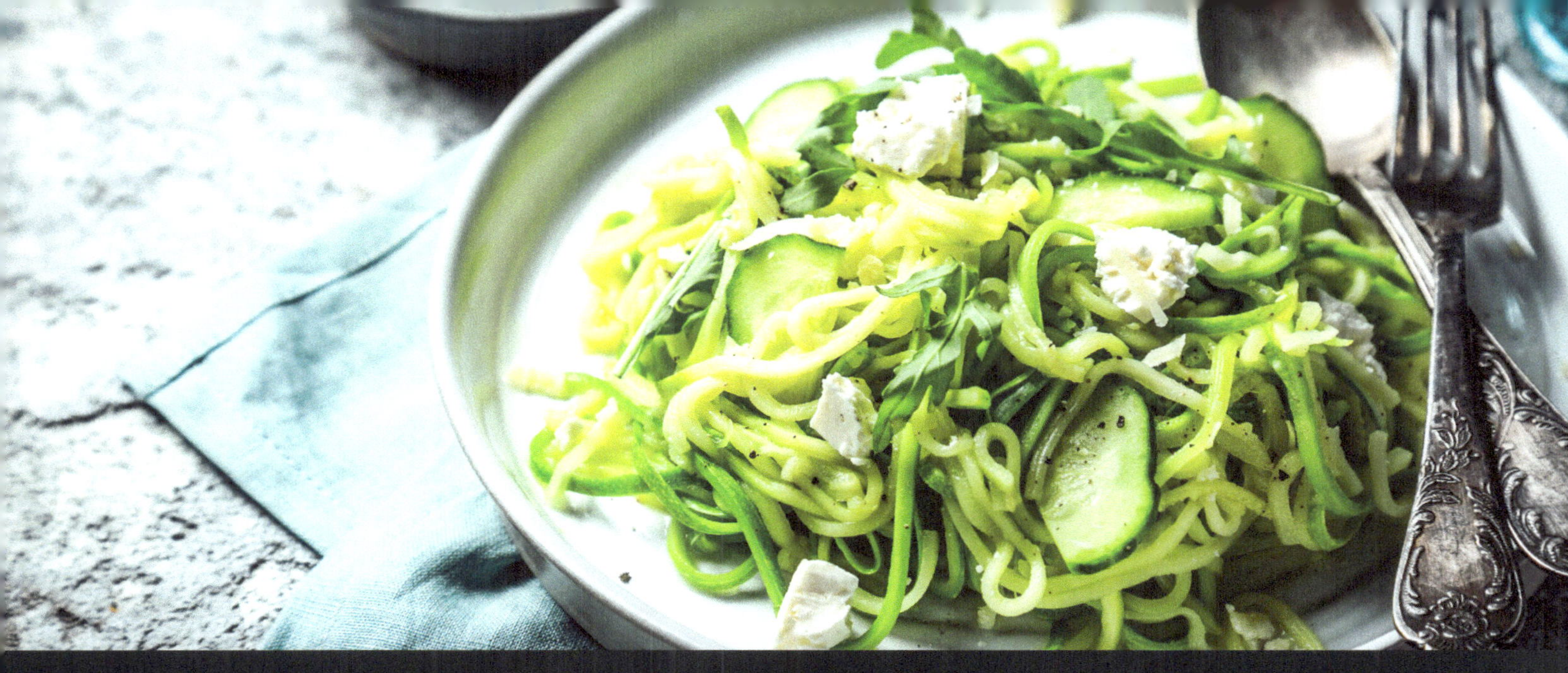

PESTO ZOODLES

Preparation Time	Cooking Time	Servings
10 min	5 min	2

Ingredients

- 2 large zucchinis, spiralized into noodles
- 1/4 cup basil pesto
- 1 cup cherry tomatoes, halved
- 1/4 cup grated Parmesan cheese
- Salt and pepper to taste

Directions

1. Heat a large skillet over medium heat. Add the zucchini noodles and prepare fcr 2-3 mins until tender-crisp.
2. Take away the skillet from the heat and add the basil pesto. Toss the zoodles until coated with the pesto.
3. Stir in the cherry tomatoes and grated Parmesan cheese. Season with salt and pepper to taste.
4. Serve the pesto zoodles warm as a light and flavorful meal.

Nutrition Information

Calories: 180 , Total Fat: 13g , Total Carbohydrates: 8g , Fiber: 3g , Protein: 8g

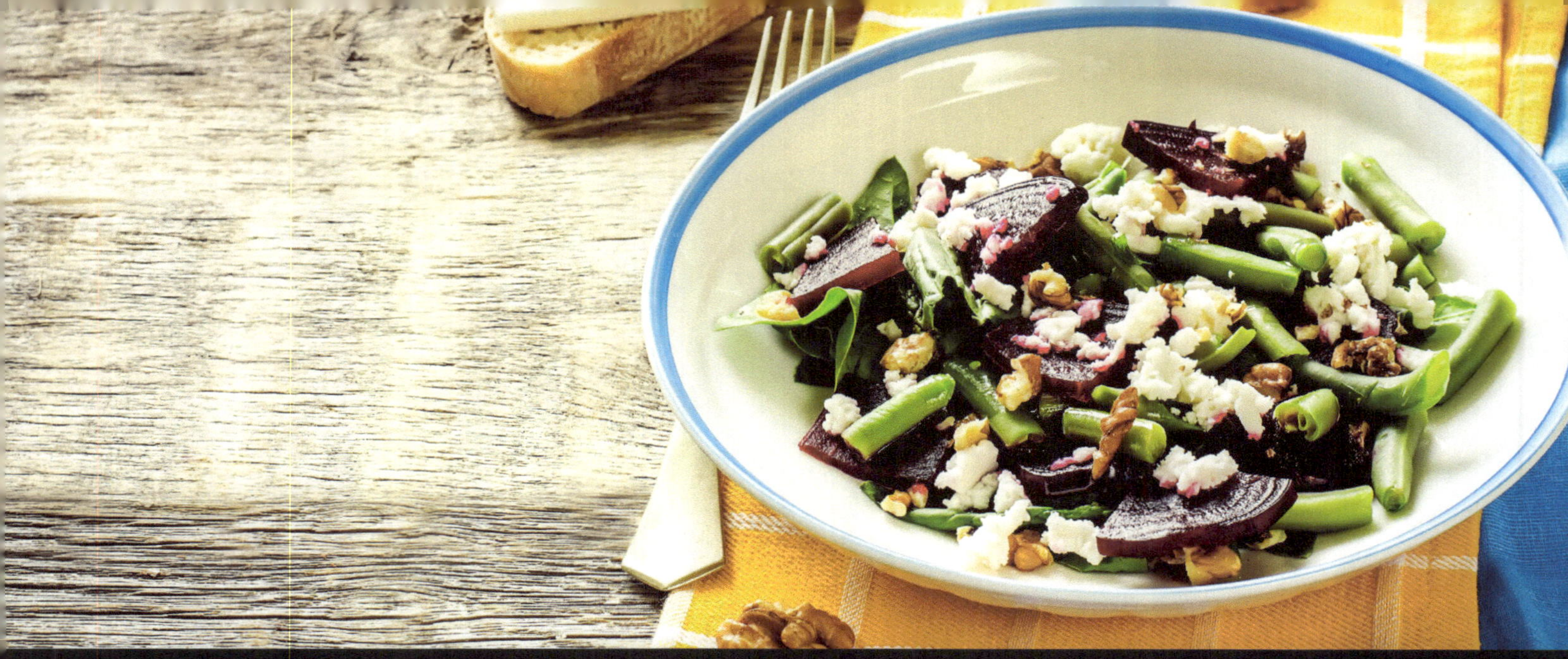

ROASTED BEET AND GOAT CHEESE SALAD

Preparation Time	Cooking Time	Servings
15 min	45 min	4

- 4 medium beets, peeled and diced
- 2 tablespoons olive oil
- Salt and pepper to taste
- 8 cups mixed salad greens
- 1/2 cup crumbled goat cheese
- 1/4 cup chopped walnuts
- 2 tablespoons balsamic vinegar
- 1 tablespoon honey

Directions

1. Set your oven's temperature to 400°F (200°C).
2. Toss the diced beets with olive oil, salt & pepper. Spread them on a baking tray and roast for 40-45 minutes or until tender.
3. Combine the roasted beets, mixed salad greens, crumbled goat cheese, and chopped walnuts in a large bowl.
4. In a bowl, whisk together the balsamic vinegar and honey. Drizzle the dressing over the salad just prior serving.

Calories: **220** , Total Fat: **15g** , Total Carbohydrates: **17g** , Fiber: **5g** , Protein: **7g**

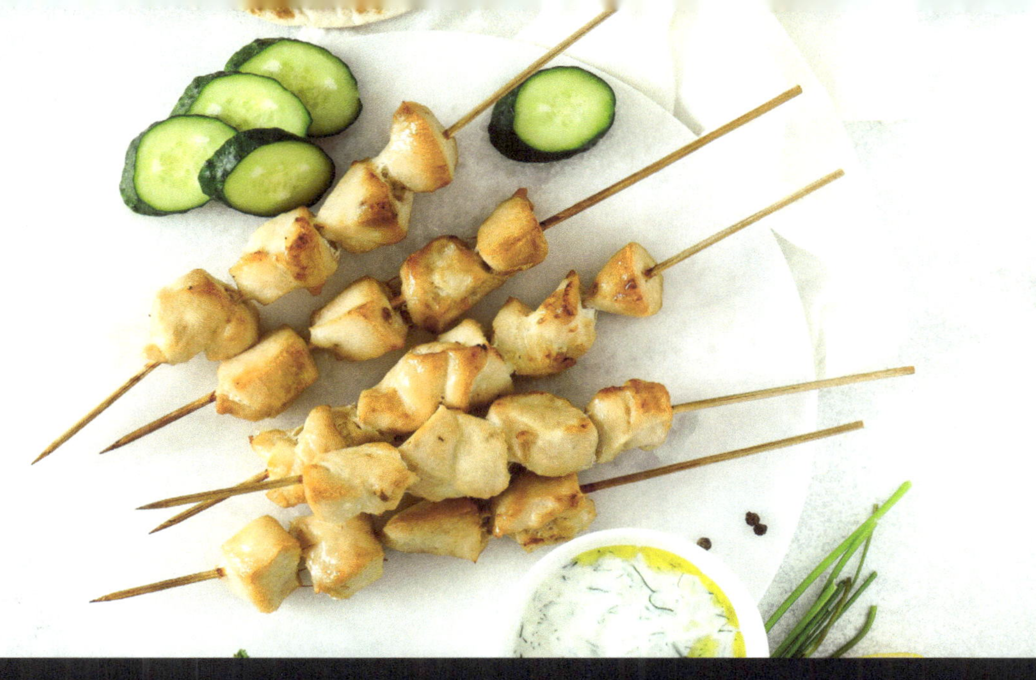

GREEK YOGURT CHICKEN KEBABS

Preparation Time	Cooking Time	Servings
20 min	20 min	4

- 1 lb. boneless, skinless breasts of chicken cut into chunks
- 1 cup plain Greek yogurt
- 2 cloves garlic, minced
- Juice of 1 lemon
- 1 tablespoon chopped fresh dill
- Salt and pepper to taste
- 1 red onion, cut into chunks
- 1 green bell pepper, cut into chunks
- 1 yellow bell pepper, cut into chunks

Directions

1. Combine the Greek yogurt, minced garlic, lemon juice, chopped dill, salt, and pepper in a bowl. Mix well.
2. Add the chicken chunks to the yogurt marinade and toss to coat. Allow it to marinate in the freezer for at least 10 mins or up to 2 hours.
3. Preheat your grill to medium heat.
4. Thread the marinated chicken, red onion, and bell peppers onto skewers.
5. Grill the chicken kebabs for 6-8 mins on each side or until the chicken is prepared.

Calories: 230 , Total Fat: 6g , Total Carbohydrates: 11g , Fiber: 2g , Protein: 33g

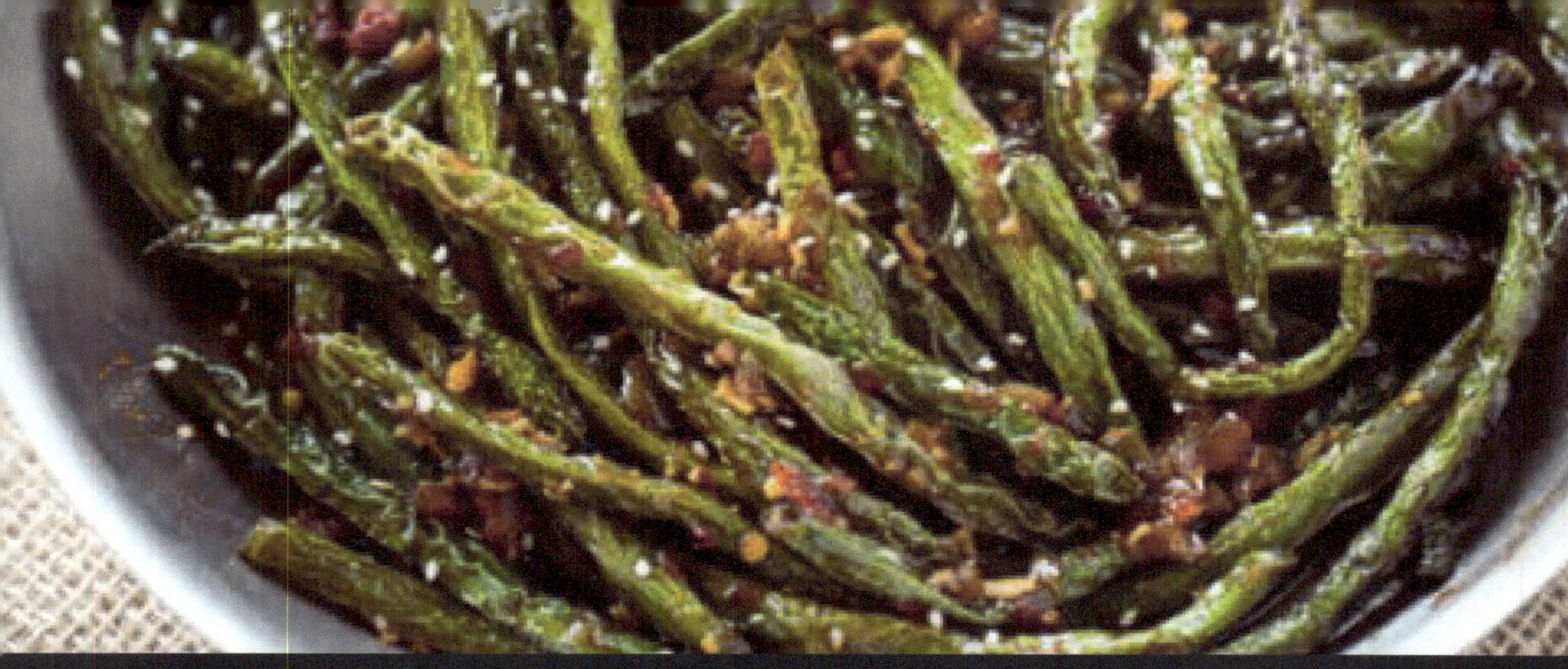

SPICY SZECHUAN GREEN BEANS

Ingredients

Preparation Time	Cooking Time	Servings
10 min	15 min	4

- 1 pound green beans, trimmed
- 2 tablespoons soy sauce
- 1 tablespoon rice vinegar
- 1 tablespoon sesame oil
- 1 tablespoon Szechuan sauce
- 1 tablespoon honey
- 2 cloves garlic, minced
- 1 teaspoon grated fresh ginger
- 1 tablespoon vegetable oil
- 2 tablespoons chopped green onions
- Sesame seeds for garnish

Directions

1. Mix a small bowl of soy sauce, rice vinegar, sesame oil, Szechuan sauce, honey, garlic, and ginger. Put away.
2. High-heat a big skillet or wok with vegetable oil. Stir-fry green beans for 4-5 minutes until crisp-tender.
3. Toss the sauce over the green beans. Cook another 2-3 minutes.
4. Add chopped green onions and sesame seeds before serving.

Nutrition Information

Calories: **110** , Total Fat: 6g , Total Carbohydrates: 12g , Fiber: 3g , Protein: 3g

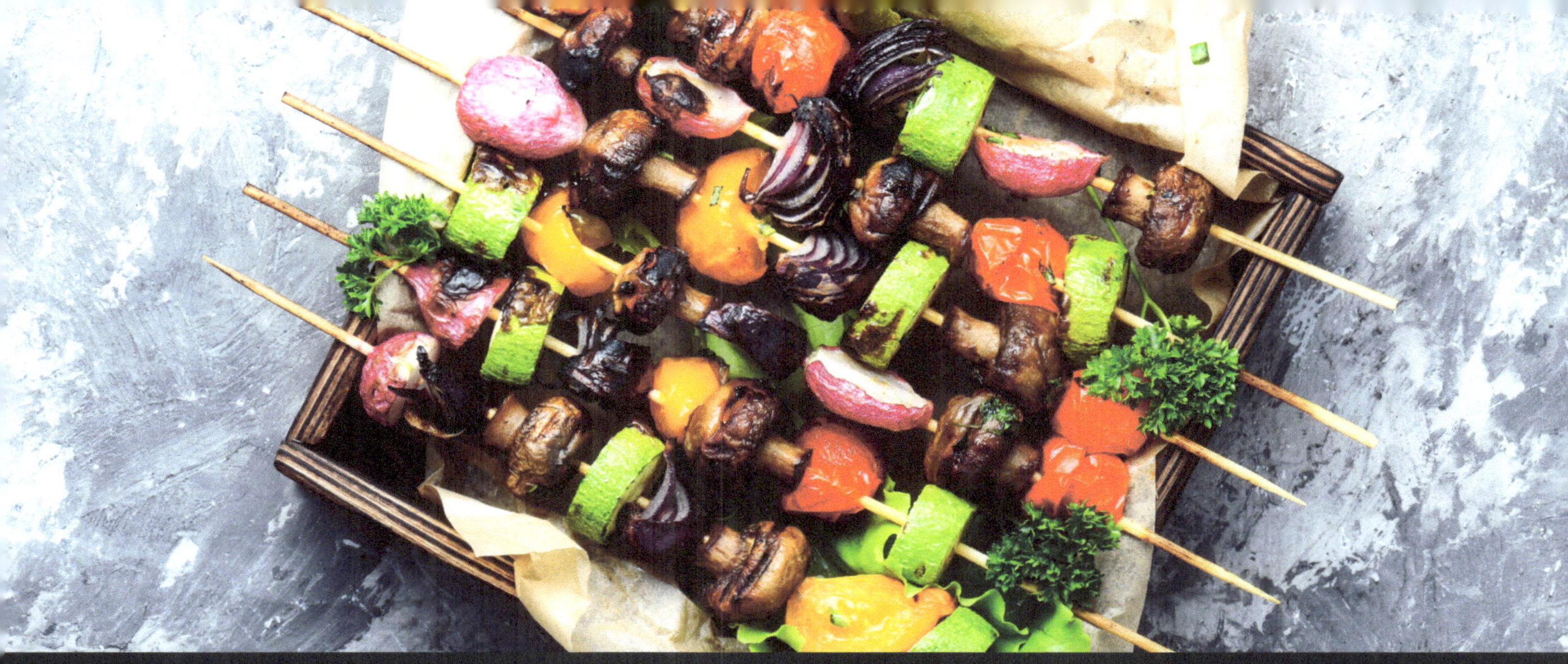

BBQ SALMON & VEGGIE SKEWERS

Preparation Time	Cooking Time	Servings
20 min	10 min	4

- 1 pound salmon fillets, cut into chunks
- 1 red bell pepper, cut into chunks
- 1 yellow bell pepper, cut into chunks
- 1 zucchini, sliced
- 1 red onion, cut into chunks
- 1/4 cup BBQ sauce
- 1 tablespoon olive oil
- Salt and pepper to taste

Directions

1. Preheat your grill to medium heat.
2. Thread the salmon chunks, bell peppers, zucchini, and red onion onto skewers.
3. Mix the BBQ sauce, olive oil, salt, and pepper in a small bowl. Brush the sauce mixture onto the skewers.
4. Grill the skewers on each side for 4-5 minutes until the salmon is cooked and the vegetables are tender.

Calories: 280 , Total Fat: 14g , Total Carbohydrates: 12gFiber: 3g
Protein: 25g

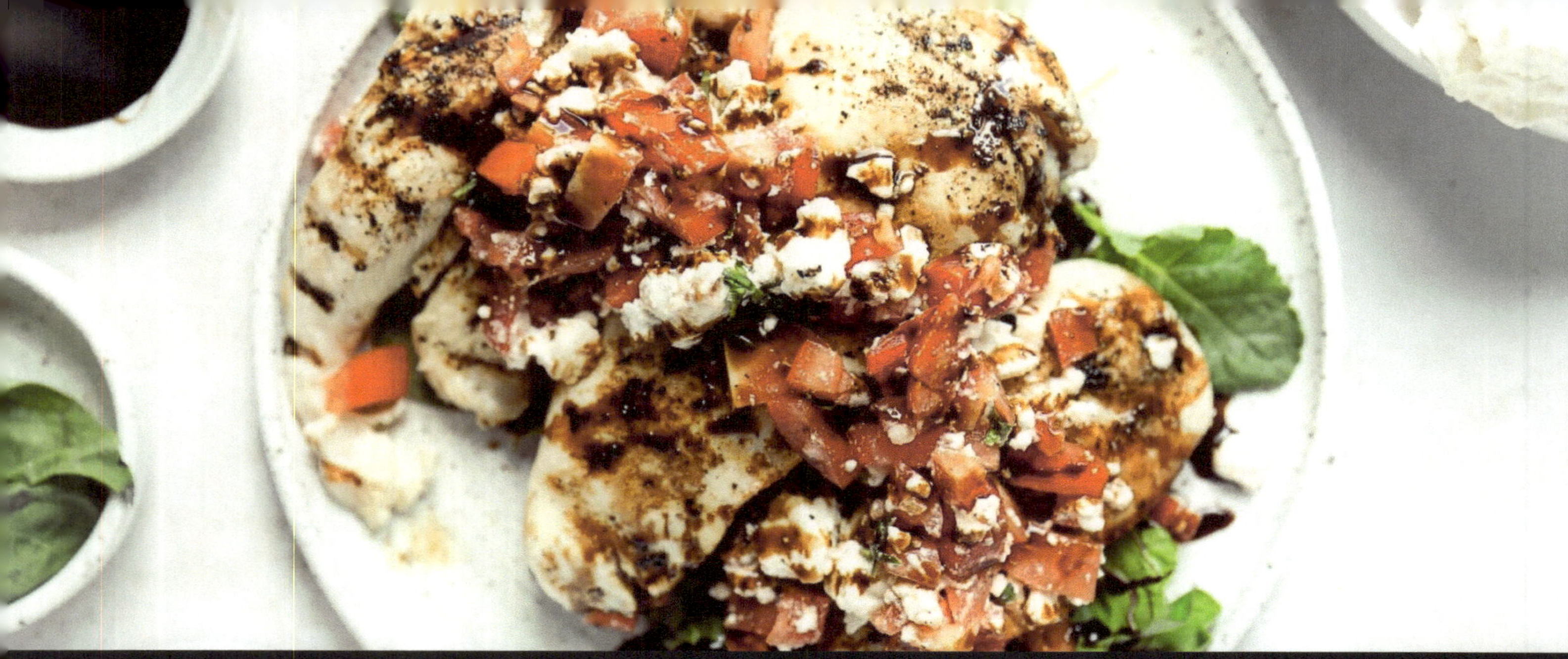

GRILLED CHICKEN BRUSCHETTA

Ingredients

Preparation Time	Cooking Time	Servings
15 min	15 min	4

- 4 boneless, skinless chicken breasts
- 2 tablespoons balsamic vinegar
- 2 tablespoons olive oil
- 2 cloves garlic, minced
- 1 teaspoon dried basil
- 1 teaspoon dried oregano
- Salt and pepper to taste
- 1 cup diced tomatoes
- 1/4 cup chopped fresh basil
- 1/4 cup grated Parmesan cheese

Directions

1. Preheat your grill to medium-high heat.
2. Whisk together the balsamic vinegar, olive oil, minced garlic, dried basil, dried oregano, salt & pepper in a small bowl. Set aside.
3. Season the chicken breasts with salt & pepper. Grill the chicken for 6-8 mins on each side until cooked.
4. Combine the diced tomatoes, chopped fresh basil, grated Parmesan cheese, and 1 tablespoon of balsamic vinegar in a separate bowl.
5. Serve the grilled chicken topped with the bruschetta mixture.

Nutrition Information

Calories: 240 , Total Fat: 9g , Total Carbohydrates: 5g , Fiber: 1g , Protein: 34g

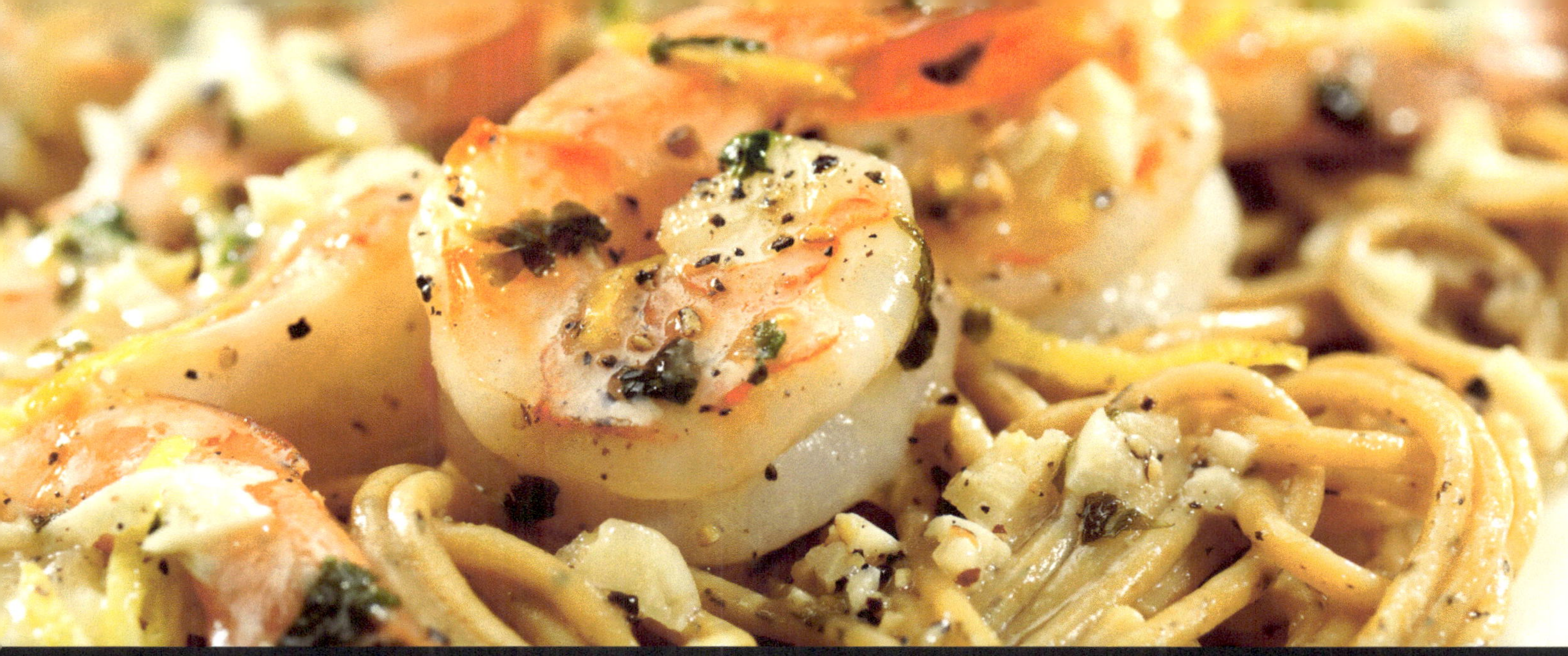

LOW-CARB SHRIMP SCAMPI

Preparation Time	Cooking Time	Servings
10 min	10 min	4

- 1 pound shrimp, peeled and deveined
- 2 tablespoons butter
- 2 cloves garlic, minced
- 1/4 cup chicken broth
- 1 tablespoon lemon juice
- 1 tablespoon chopped fresh parsley
- Salt and pepper to taste
- Zucchini noodles or spaghetti squash for serving

Directions

1. In a big non-stick skillet, melt the butter over moderate heat; after adding the garlic, mince and cook it for approximately a minute.
2. until it smells wonderful.
3. Cook shrimp in the skillet for 2-3 minutes per side until pink and done. Set shrimp aside from skillet.
4. Chicken broth and lime juice into the skillet. Simmer for 2 minutes, scraping the skillet to blend flavors.
5. Toss shrimp with sauce in a skillet. Add chopped parsley and salt and pepper.
6. Serve the shrimp scampi over zucchini noodles or spaghetti squash.

Nutrition Information

Calories: 160 , Total Fat: 7g , Total Carbohydrates: 3g , Fiber: 0g , Protein: 22g

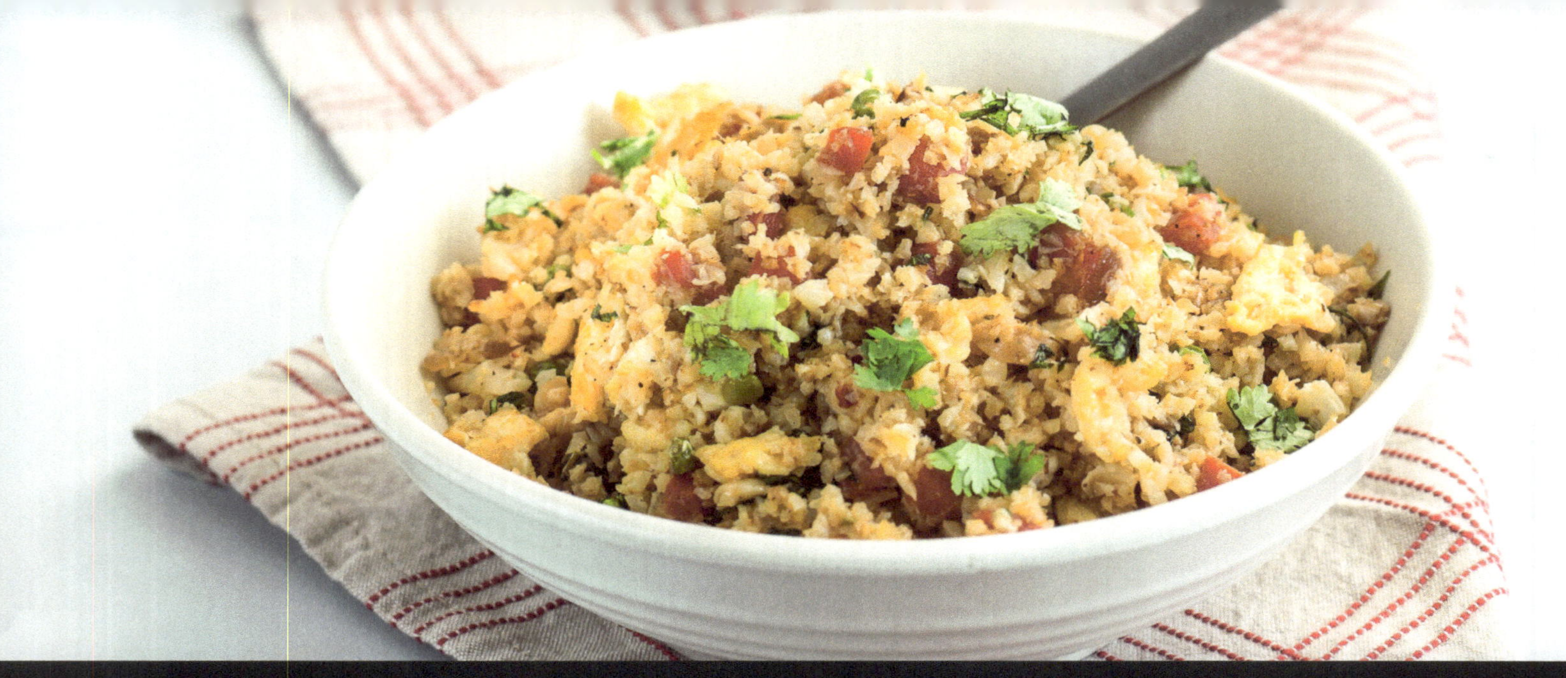

SPICED CAULIFLOWER RICE

Preparation Time	Cooking Time	Servings
10 min	10 min	4

- 1 head cauliflower, riced (or use pre-packaged cauliflower rice)
- 1 tablespoon olive oil
- 1/2 teaspoon ground cumin
- 1/2 teaspoon paprika
- 1/4 teaspoon turmeric
- Salt and pepper to taste
- Chopped fresh cilantro for garnish

Directions

1. Warm the olive oil in a big skillet over normal heat. Add the riced cauliflower and cook for 5 minutes, stirring occasionally.
2. Sprinkle the ground cumin, paprika, turmeric, salt, and pepper over the cauliflower rice. Stir well to combine and cook for another 5 minutes.
3. Garnish with chopped fresh cilantro before serving.

Nutrition Information

Calories: 50, Total Fat: 3g , Total Carbohydrates: 5g , Fiber: 2g , Protein: 2g

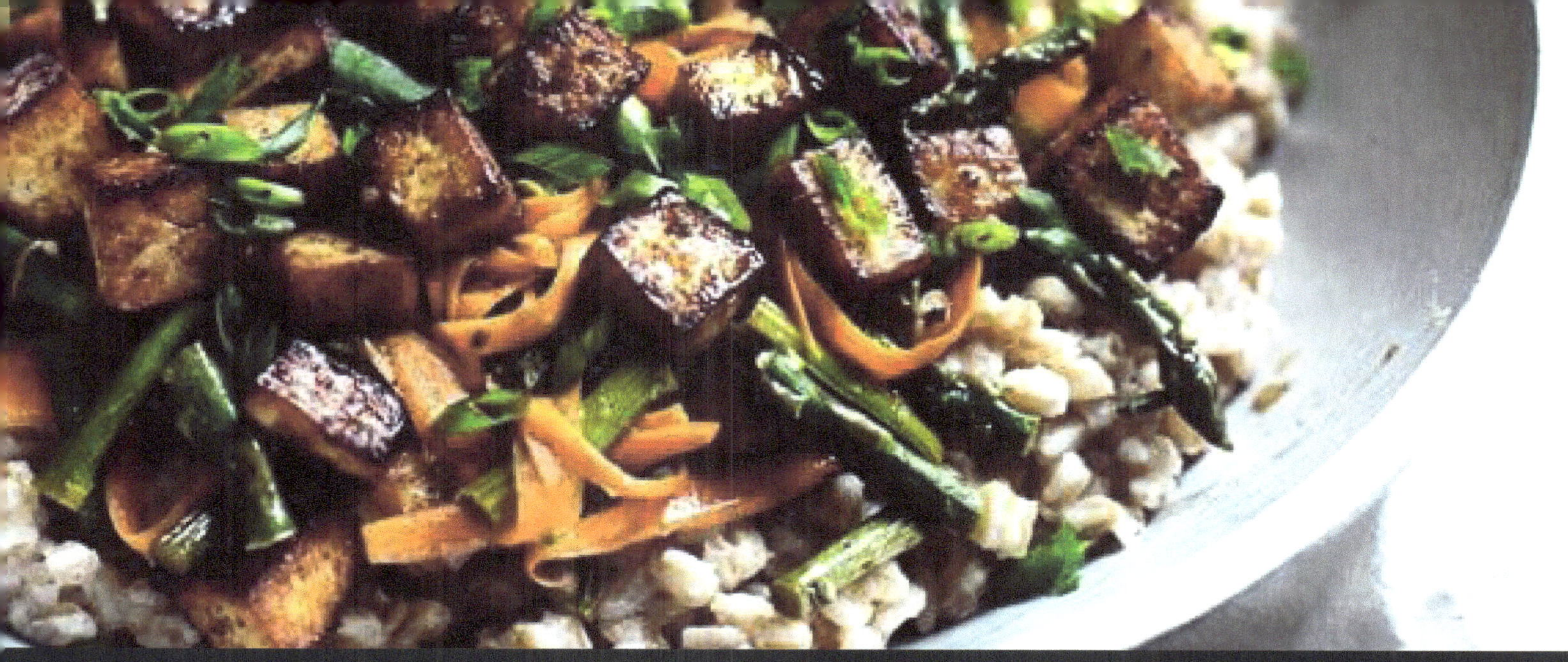

GINGER SOY TOFU STIR-FRY

Preparation Time 15 min	Cooking Time 10 min	Servings 4

- 1 block extra-firm tofu, drained and pressed
- 2 tablespoons soy sauce
- 1 tablespoon rice vinegar
- 1 tablespoon honey
- 1 tablespoon grated fresh ginger
- 2 cloves garlic, minced
- 1 tablespoon vegetable oil
- 2 cups mixed stir-fried vegetables (such as bell peppers, broccoli, and snap peas)
- 2 green onions, chopped
- Sesame seeds for garnish

Directions

1. Cut the pressed tofu into cubes.
2. Mix a bowl of soy sauce, rice vinegar, honey, grated ginger, and minced garlic. Set aside.
3. Medium-heat a large skillet or wok with vegetable oil. After 5 or 6 minutes, add the tofu cubes and fry them until they are golden brown on all sides. Set aside.
4. the skillet-cooked tofu.
5. Stir-fry veggies and green onions in the same skillet. Cook for three to four mins or until the vegetables reach a crisp-tender consistency.
6. Pour the soy sauce blending over the tofu and vegetables. Toss everything with sauce.
7. Cook for one to two minutes, stirring occasionally, until the sauce is hot.
8. Garnish with sesame seeds before serving.

Calories: 180 , Total Fat: 8g , Total Carbohydrates: 17g , Fiber: 3g , Protein: 12g

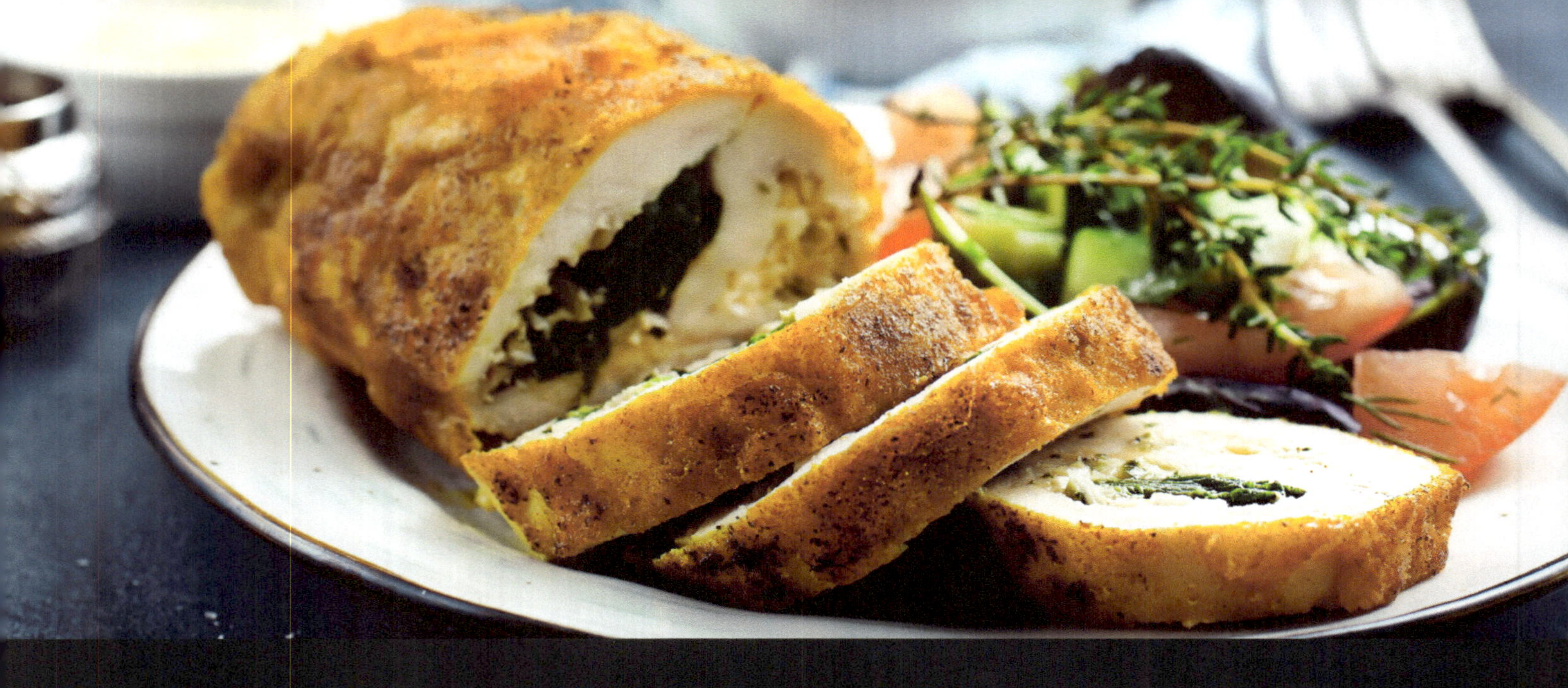

FETA STUFFED CHICKEN BREASTS

Preparation Time	Cooking Time	Servings
15 min	25 min	4

- 4 boneless, skinless chicken breasts
- 1/4 cup crumbled feta cheese
- 1/4 cup chopped sun-dried tomatoes
- 1 tablespoon chopped fresh basil
- 1 tablespoon olive oil
- Salt and pepper to taste

Directions

1. Adjust your oven's temperature to 375°F (190°C).
2. Slice a pocket into each chicken breast, careful not to cut through.
3. Mix the crumbled feta cheese, sun-dried tomatoes chopped fresh basil in a small bowl.
4. Spread the feta mixture on each chicken breast and roll it up, pressing the seams to close.
5. Salt and pepper the chicken breasts before stuffing them.
6. Warm olive oil in an oven-safe skillet on medium-high. Brown the chicken breasts for 3–4 minutes per side.
7. Place the cast iron pan in a heated oven and bake for 15 to 20 mins to cook the chicken.

Nutrition Information

Calories: 250 , Total Fat: 9g , Total Carbohydrates: 2g , Fiber: 0g , Protein: 37g

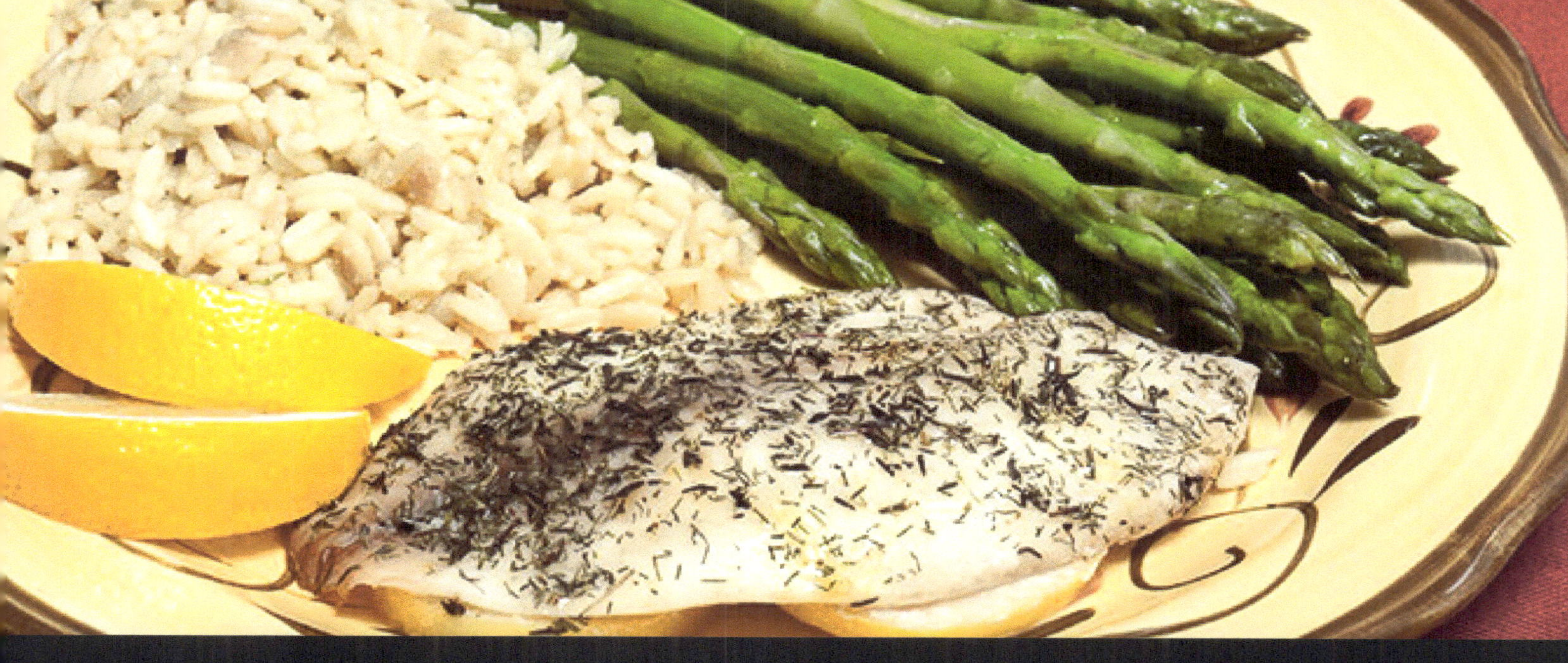

LEMON DILL HADDOCK

Preparation Time	Cooking Time	Servings
10 min	15 min	4

Ingredients

- 4 haddock fillets
- 2 tablespoons olive oil
- Juice of 1 lemon
- 1 tablespoon chopped fresh dill
- Salt and pepper to taste
- Lemon wedges for serving

Directions

1. Set your oven's temperature to 400°F (200°C).
2. Place the haddock fillets on a baking sheet lined with parchment paper.
3. Whisk together the olive oil, lime juice, chopped dill, salt, and pepper in a bowl. Drizzle the mixture over the haddock fillets, spreading it evenly.
4. Prepare in the oven for 12-15 mins or until the fish is prepared and flakes easily with a fork.
5. Serve the lemon dill haddock with lemon wedges on the side.

Nutrition Information

Calories: 180 , Total Fat: 9g , Total Carbohydrates: 1g , Fiber: 0g , Protein: 23g

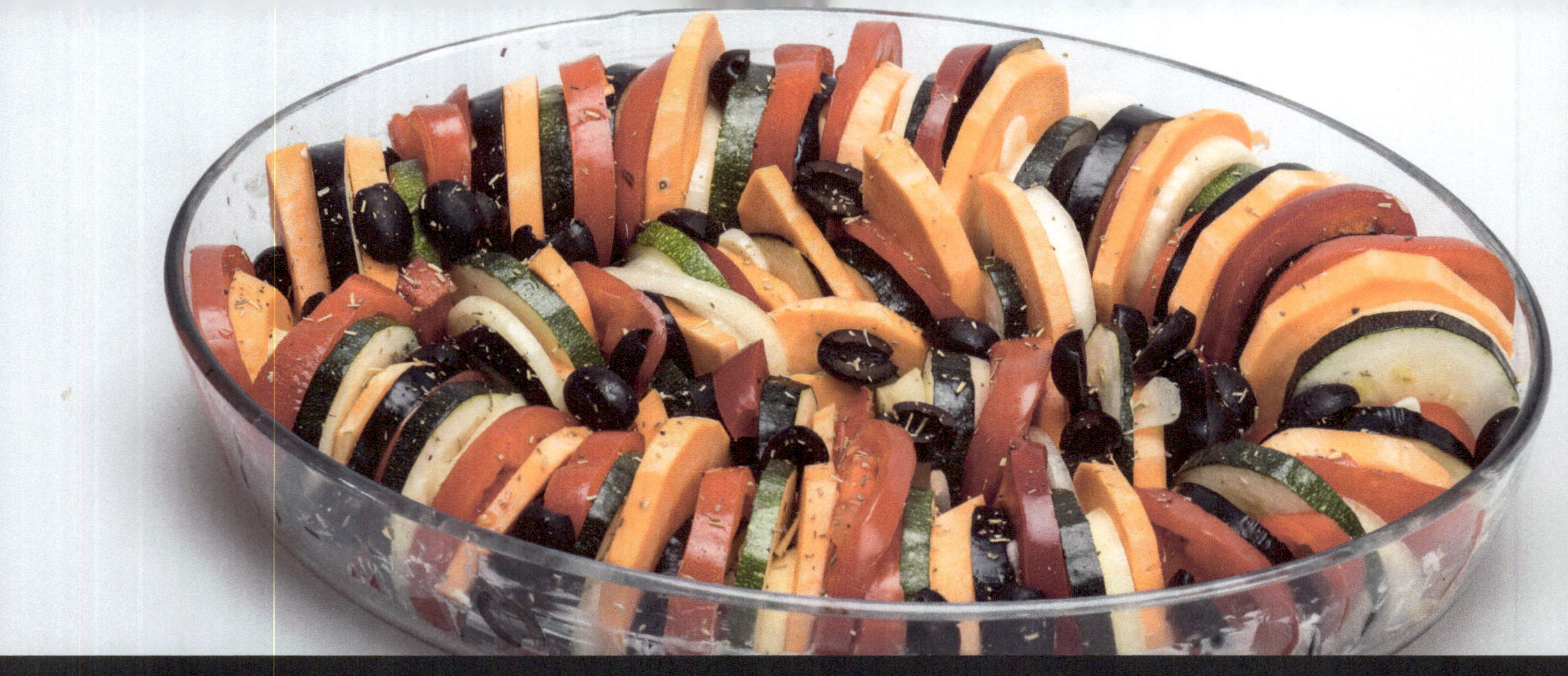

PROVENÇAL RATATOUILLE

Preparation Time	Cooking Time	Servings
20 min	40 min	6

Ingredients

- 2 tablespoons olive oil
- 1 onion, diced
- 2 cloves garlic, minced
- 1 eggplant, diced
- 1 zucchini, diced
- 1 yellow squash, diced
- 1 red bell pepper, diced
- 1 yellow bell pepper, diced
- 1 can diced tomatoes
- 1 tablespoon tomato paste
- 1 teaspoon dried thyme
- 1 teaspoon dried oregano
- Salt and pepper to taste
- Chopped fresh basil for garnish

Directions

1. Medium-heat olive oil in a big pot or Dutch oven. Add onion and garlic. About 5 minutes should be enough time for the onion to become clear.
2. Add diced eggplant, zucchini, yellow squash, and red and yellow bell peppers to the pot. Ten minutes, stirring periodically.
3. Stir in the diced tomatoes, tomato paste, dried thyme, oregano, salt, and pepper. Cover the saucepan and cook on low for 25–30 minutes until the vegetables are cooked.
4. Garnish with chopped fresh basil before serving.

Nutrition Information

Calories: 120 , Total Fat: 6g , Total Carbohydrates: 15g , Fiber: 5g , Protein: 3g

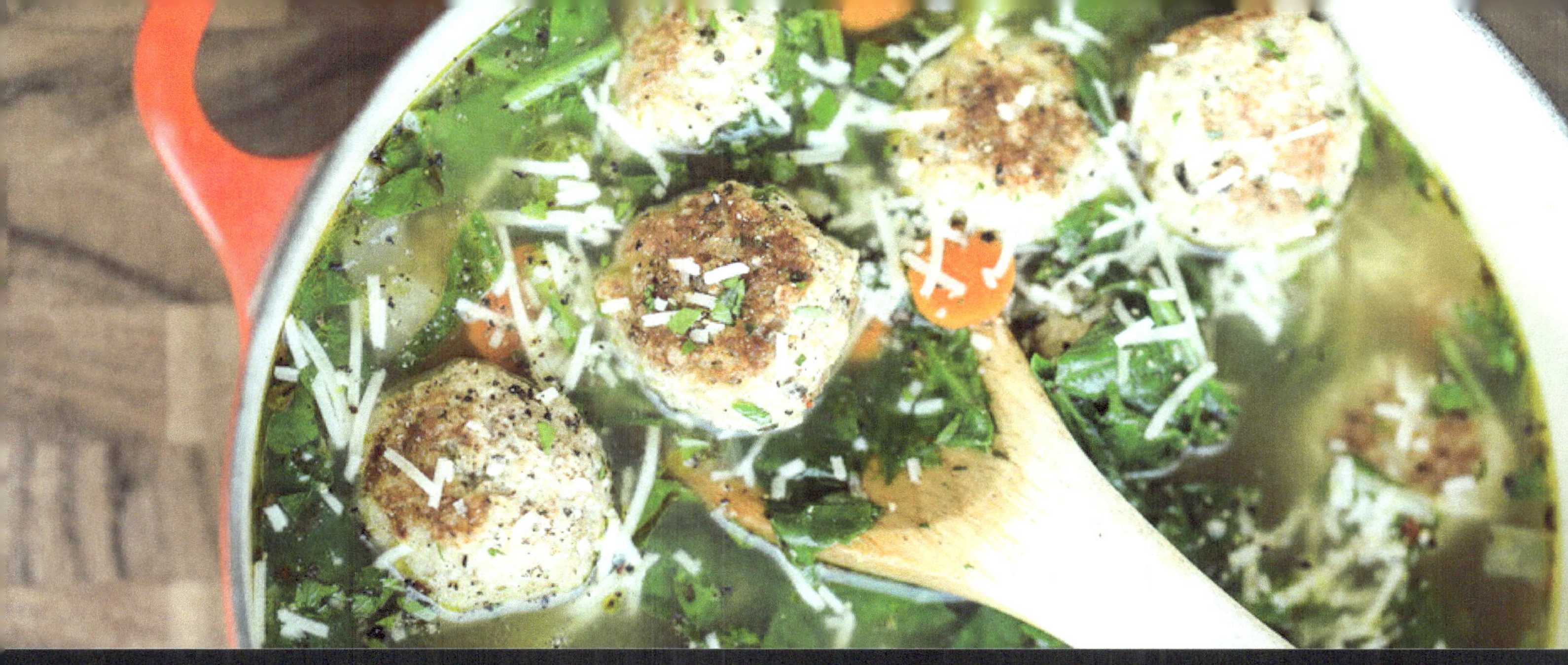

TURKEY MEATBALL SPINACH SOUP

Ingredients

Preparation Time	Cooking Time	Servings
20 min	30 min	6

- 1 pound ground turkey
- 1/4 cup breadcrumbs
- 1/4 cup grated Parmesan cheese
- 1/4 cup chopped fresh parsley
- 1/4 cup chopped onion
- 2 cloves garlic, minced
- 1 egg
- 1 teaspoon dried oregano
- Salt and pepper to taste
- 1 tablespoon olive oil
- 4 cups chicken broth
- 2 cups fresh spinach
- 1 cup chopped carrots
- 1 cup chopped celery

Directions

1. Combine the ground turkey, breadcrumbs, grated Parmesan cheese, chopped parsley, chopped onion, minced garlic, egg, dried oregano, salt, and pepper in a bowl. Mix well and shape into meatballs.
2. Medium-heat olive oil in a big pot. Add the meatballs and cook for about 5 minutes, until they are cooked on all sides. Set meatballs aside.
3. Add chicken broth, fresh spinach, diced carrots, and chopped celery to the pot. Please take it to a boil, then turn down the heat and let it cook for 15 minutes.
4. Put the meatballs back in the pot and let them cook for 10 minutes or until the meatballs are done and the veggies are soft.

Nutrition Information

Calories: 200 , Total Fat: 9g , Total Carbohydrates: 9g , Fiber: 2g , Protein: 21g

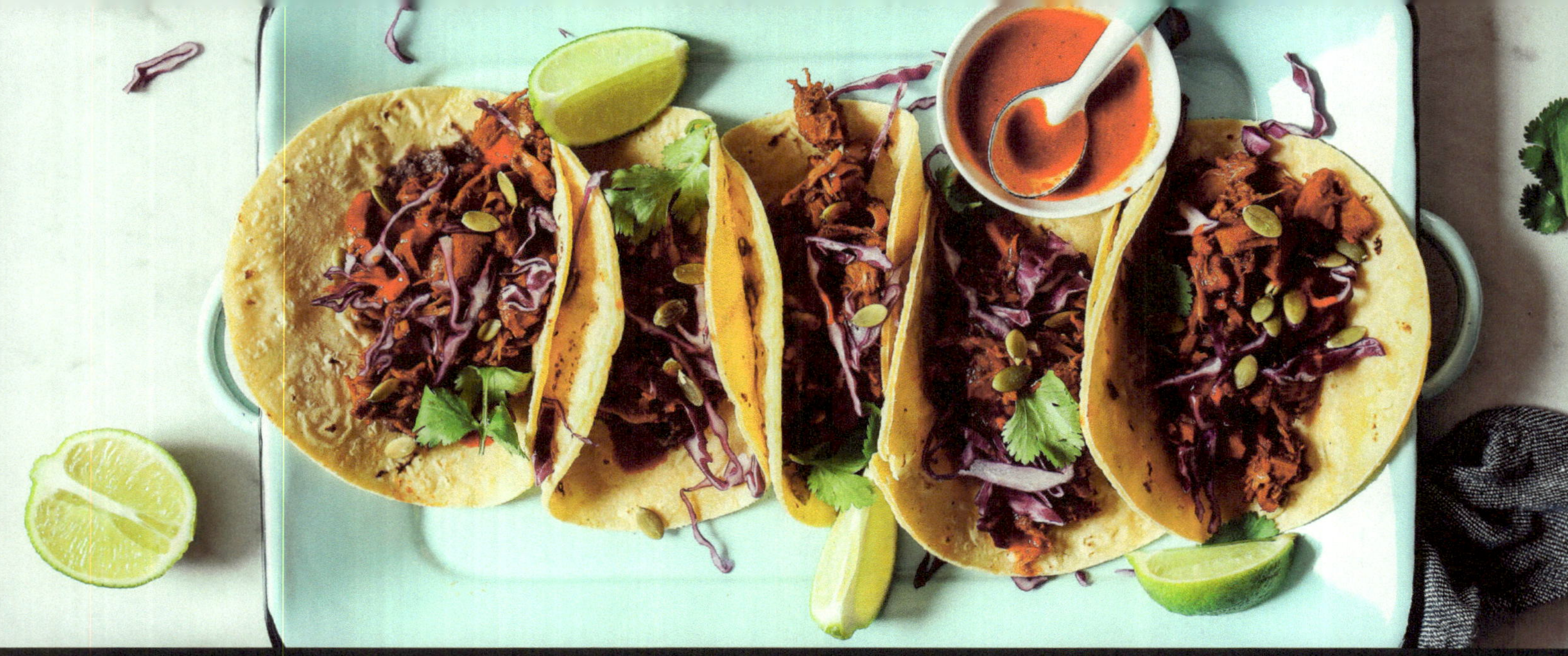

SPICY BBQ JACKFRUIT TACOS

Preparation Time	Cooking Time	Servings
20 min	25 min	4

- 2 cans of young jackfruit in water or brine
- 1/2 cup BBQ sauce
- 1 tablespoon olive oil
- 1/2 teaspoon smoked paprika
- 1/2 teaspoon chili powder
- Salt and pepper to taste
- 8 small corn tortillas
- 1 cup shredded lettuce
- 1/2 cup diced tomatoes
- 1/4 cup diced red onion
- Fresh cilantro for garnish

Directions

1. Drain and rinse the jackfruit. Shred the jackfruit by hand or fork until it is very small.
2. Medium-heat olive oil in a skillet. Shredded jackfruit, smoked paprika, chili powder, salt, and pepper. Five minutes, stirring periodically.
3. Stir jackfruit with BBQ sauce. For 10 minutes, cook and flavor the jackfruit with BBQ.
4. Dry skillet or microwave the corn tortillas.
5. Assemble the tacos by placing a scoop of BBQ jackfruit on each tortilla. Top with shredded lettuce, tomatoes, red onion, and fresh cilantro.

Nutrition Information

Calories: 250 , Total Fat: 6g , Total Carbohydrates: 47g , Fiber: 10g , Protein: 4g

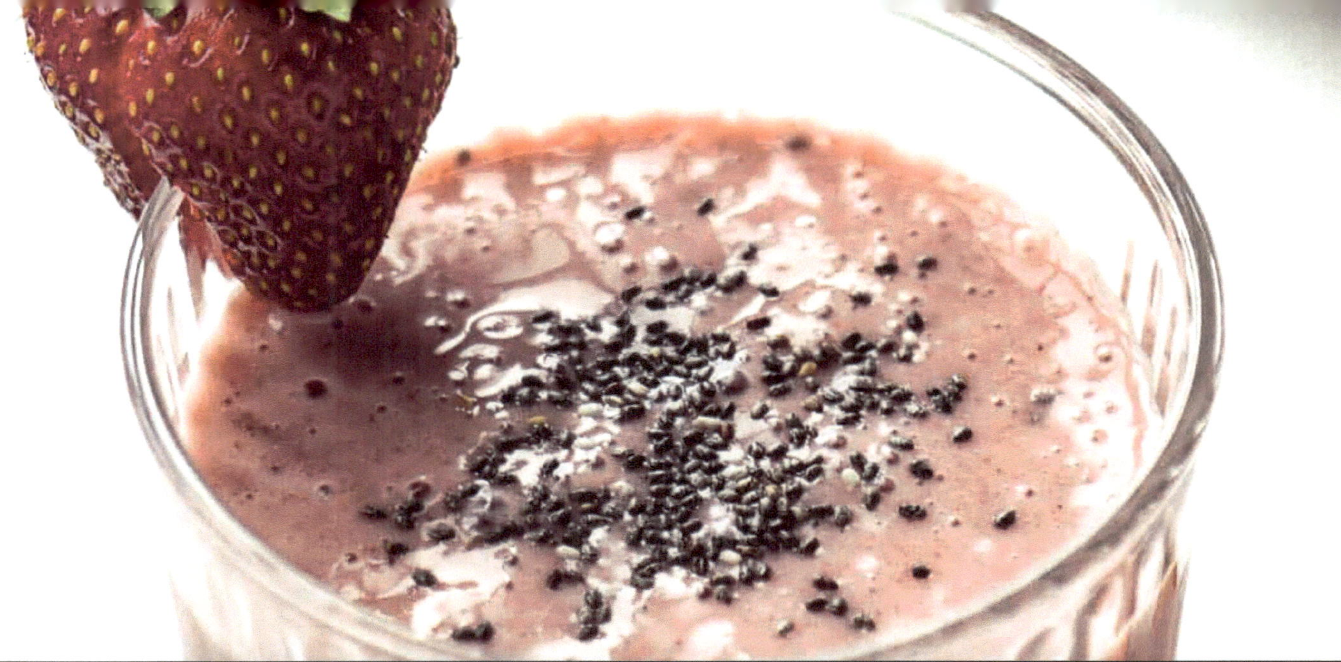

STRAWBERRY CHIA SMOOTHIE

Preparation Time	Cooking Time	Servings
5 min	0 min	2

- 1 cup frozen strawberries
- 1 ripe banana
- 1 cup unsweetened almond milk
- 1 tablespoon chia seeds
- 1 tablespoon honey or maple syrup (optional)
- Fresh mint leaves, for garnish

Directions

1. If desired, blend the frozen strawberries, ripe banana, almond milk, chia seeds, and honey or maple syrup.
2. Blend until smooth and creamy.
3. Pour the strawberry chia smoothie into glasses and garnish with fresh mint leaves.

Calories: 120 , Total Fat: 3g , Total Carbohydrates: 23g , Fiber: 7g , Protein: 2g

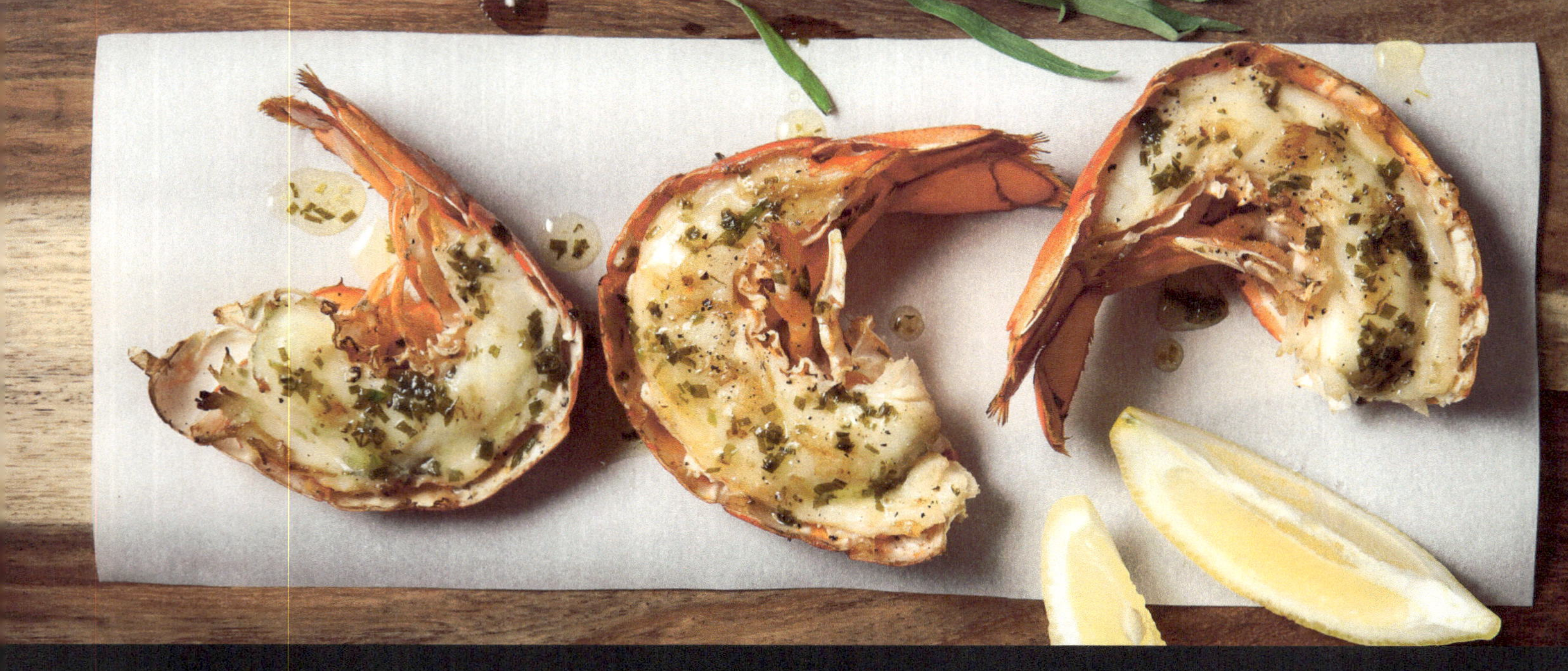

GRILLED LOBSTER TAILS

Preparation Time	Cooking Time	Servings
10 min	10 min	2

- 2 lobster tails
- 2 tablespoons melted butter
- 1 tablespoon lemon juice
- 1 teaspoon chopped fresh parsley
- Salt and pepper to taste

Directions

1. Preheat your grill to moderate heat.
2. Use kitchen shears to trim the top shell off the lobster tails, stopping at the base of the tail.
3. Gently spread the shell open to expose the meat.
4. Mix the melted butter, lemon juice, chopped parsley, salt, and pepper in a small bowl.
5. Brush the butter blending over the lobster meat.
6. Place the lobster tails on the grill, meat side down, and cook for 5 minutes.
7. Flip the lobster tails and continue grilling for another 5 minutes or until the meat is opaque and cooked through.

Nutrition Information

Calories: 180 , Total Fat: 10g , Total Carbohydrates: 2g , Fiber: 0g , Protein: 20g

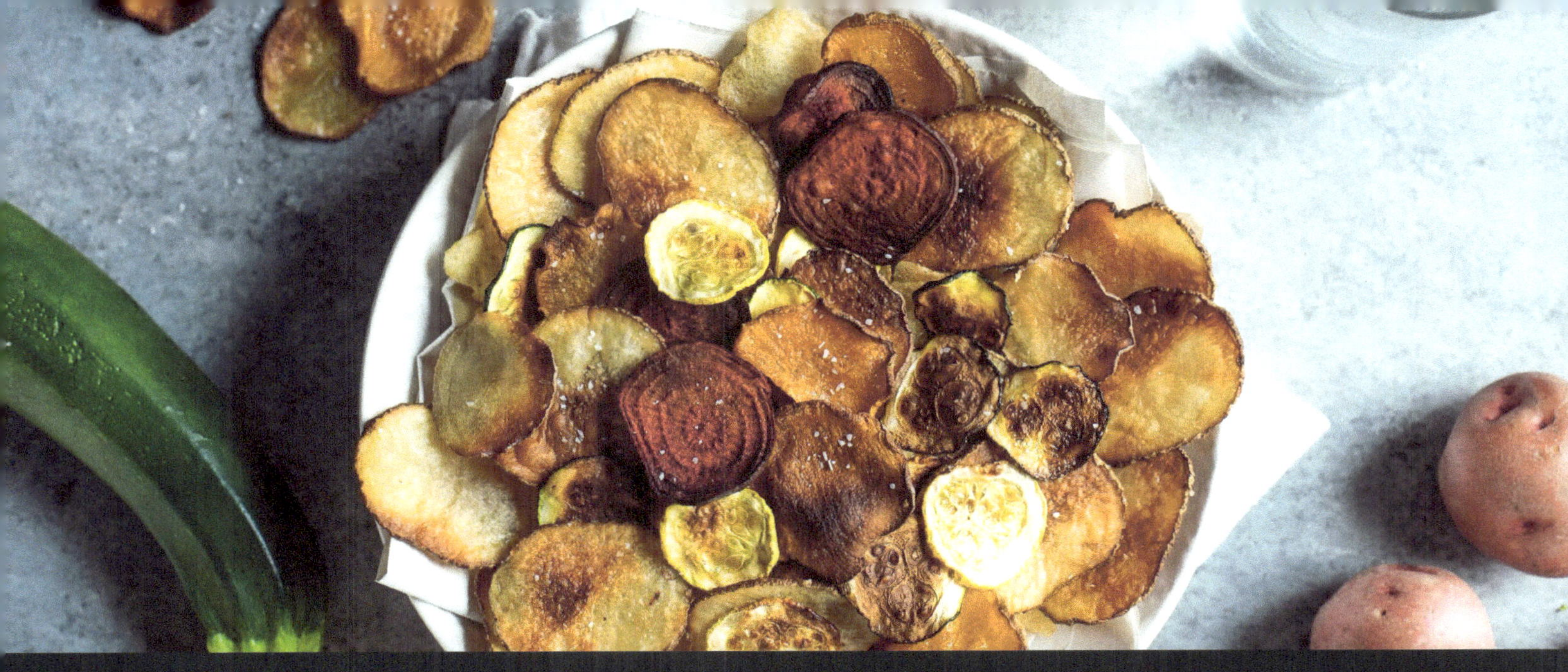

BAKED VEGGIE CHIPS

Preparation Time	Cooking Time	Servings
10 min	20 min	4

Ingredients

- 2 large sweet potatoes
- 2 large beets
- 2 tablespoons olive oil
- Salt and pepper to taste

Directions

1. Adjust your oven to 375°F (190°C).
2. Slice the sweet potatoes and beets into thin rounds using a mandoline slicer or a sharp knife.
3. Place the sliced sweet potatoes and beets in separate bowls. Drizzle each with 1 tbsp of olive oil, salt, and pepper. Toss to coat.
4. Arrange the sweet potato and beet slices on separate baking sheets in a single layer.
5. Prepare in the oven for 15-20 mins or until the chips are crispy and golden.
6. Allow the chips to cool before serving.

Nutrition Information

Calories: 120 , Total Fat: 5g , Total Carbohydrates: 17g , Fiber: 3g , Protein: 2g

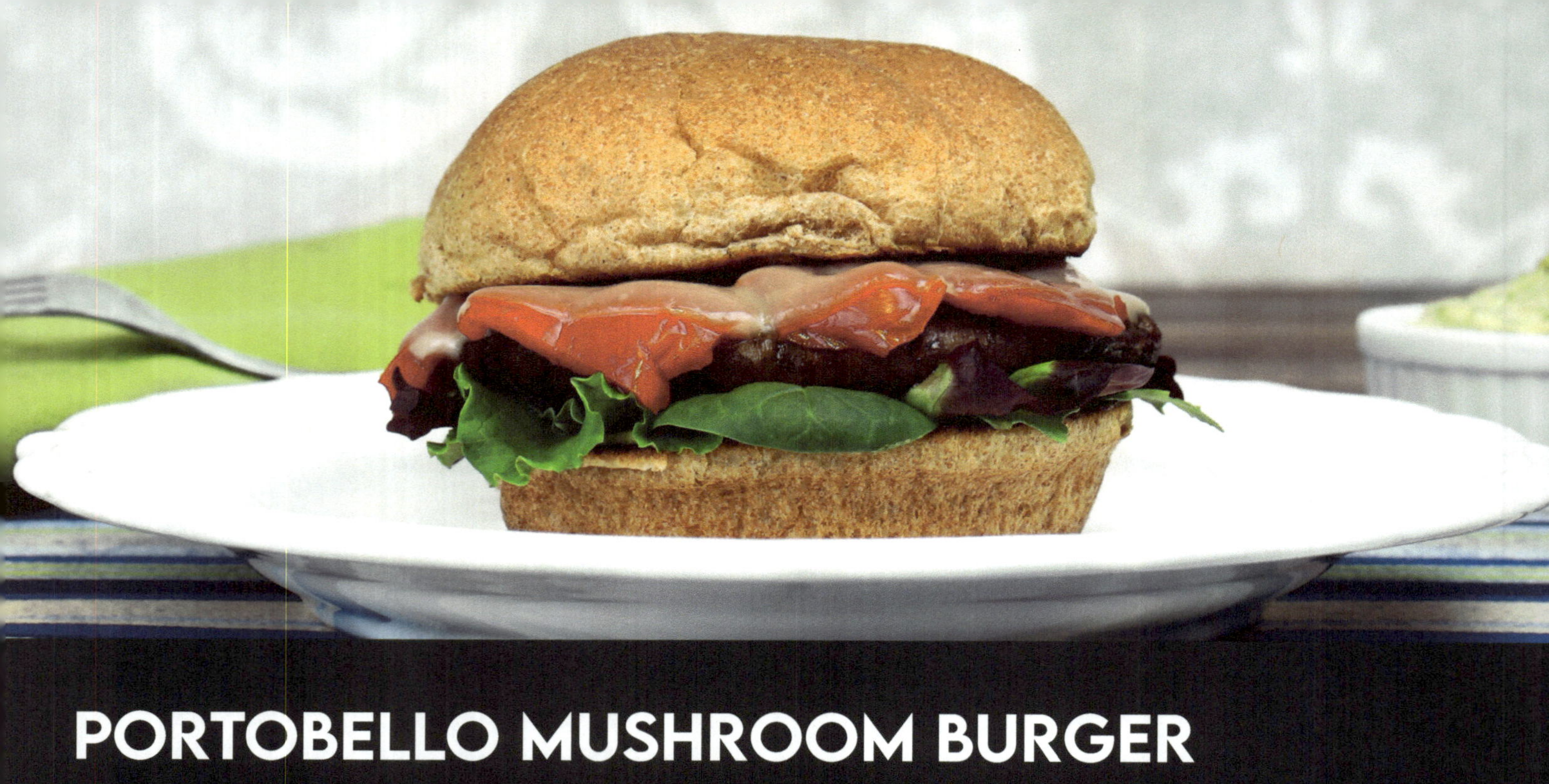

PORTOBELLO MUSHROOM BURGER

Preparation Time	Cooking Time	Servings
15 min	10 min	2

- 2 large Portobello mushroom caps
- 2 tablespoons balsamic vinegar
- 1 tablespoon olive oil
- 1 teaspoon soy sauce
- 1/2 teaspoon garlic powder
- Salt and pepper to taste
- 2 whole wheat burger buns
- Toppings of your choice (lettuce, tomato, onion, avocado, etc.)

Directions

1. Preheat your grill or grill pan to moderate heat.
2. Mix the balsamic vinegar, olive oil, soy sauce, garlic powder, salt & pepper in a bowl.
3. Brush the mushroom caps with the balsamic mixture, coating both sides.
4. Grill the mushroom caps for 4-5 minutes on each side or until tender and juicy.
5. Put the burger buns on the grill and let them toast for a few minutes.
6. Assemble the Portobello mushroom burgers with your toppings on the toasted buns.

Calories: 180 , Total Fat: 7g , Total Carbohydrates: 27g , Fiber: 6g , Protein: 6g

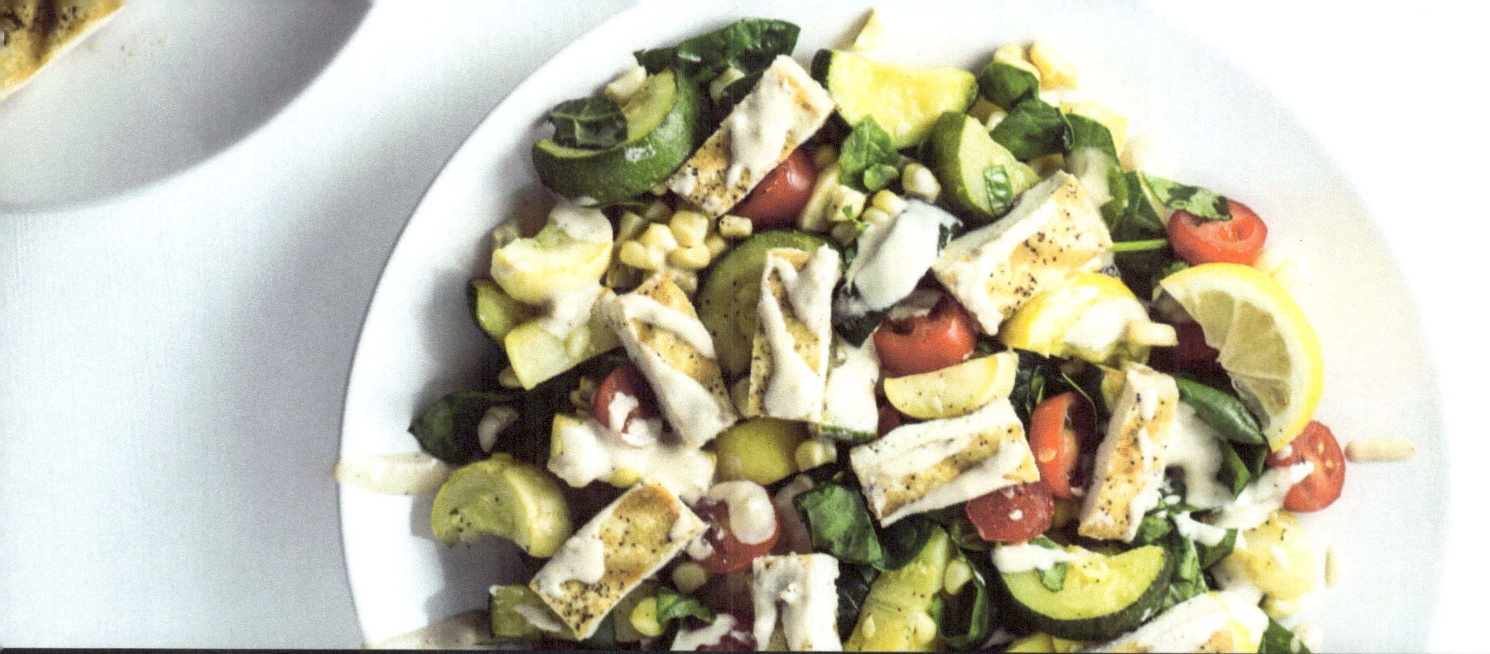

GRILLED TOFU & VEGGIE SALAD

Preparation Time	Cooking Time	Servings
20 min	10 min	2

- 1 block firm tofu, drained and pressed
- 2 tablespoons soy sauce
- 1 tablespoon olive oil
- 1 tablespoon lemon juice
- 1 teaspoon Dijon mustard
- 1 clove garlic, minced
- Salt and pepper to taste
- 4 cups mixed salad greens
- 1 cup cherry tomatoes, halved
- 1/2 cup sliced cucumber
- 1/4 cup sliced red onion
- 2 tbsp fresh herbs chopped (such as basil, parsley, or cilantro)

Directions

1. Preheat your grill to medium-high heat.
2. Make pieces or cubes out of the pressed tofu.
3. Whisk together the soy sauce, olive oil, lemon juice, Dijon mustard, minced garlic, salt, and pepper in a small bowl.
4. Brush the tofu with the marinade, reserving some for the dressing.
5. Grill the tofu on each side for 3-4 minutes or until browned and heated.
6. Combine the mixed salad greens, cherry tomatoes, sliced cucumber, red onion, and chopped fresh herbs in a large bowl.
7. Toss the salad with the reserved marinade to coat evenly.
8. Serve the grilled tofu on top of the salad.

Calories: 240 , Total Fat: 12g , Total Carbohydrates: 18g , Fiber: 5g , Protein: 19g

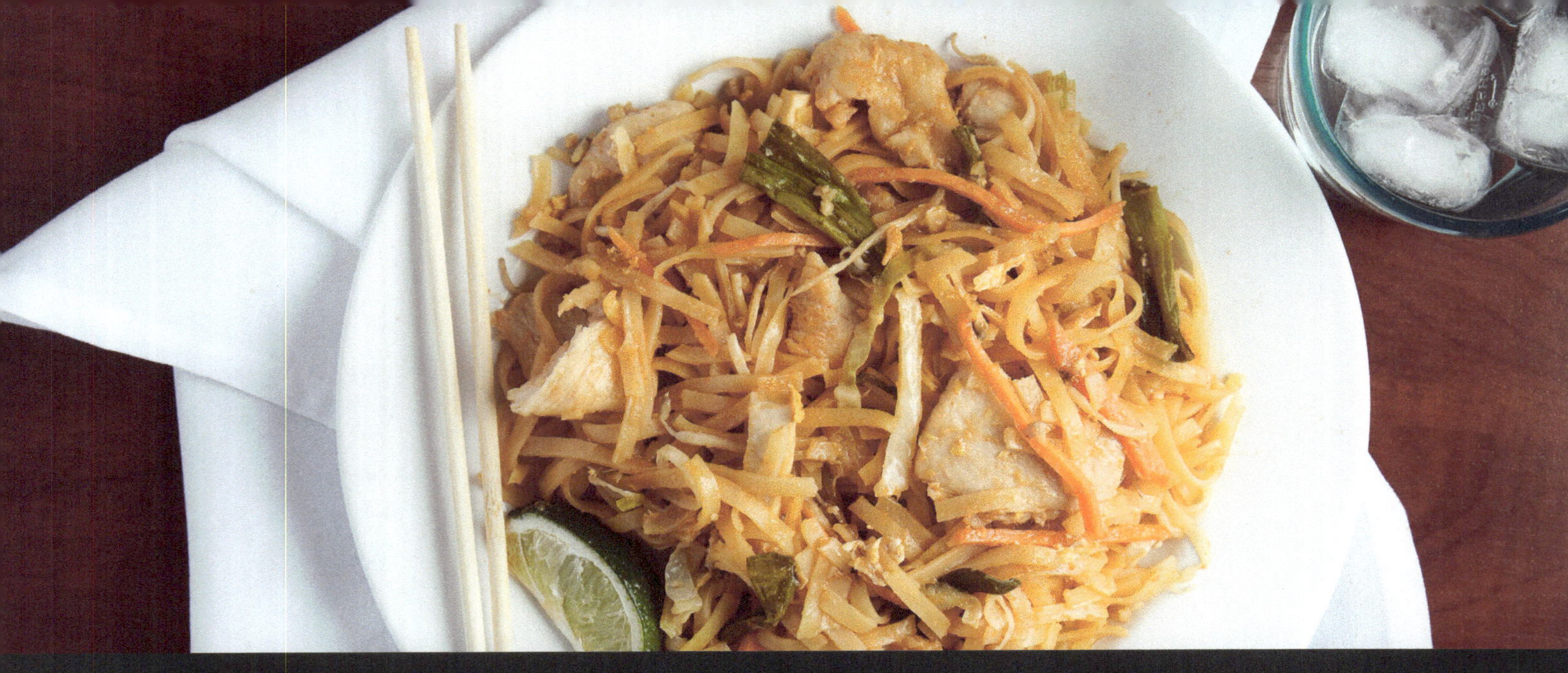

LOW-CARB CHICKEN PAD THAI

Preparation Time	Cooking Time	Servings
20 min	15 min	4

- 2 medium zucchinis, spiralized into noodles
- 2 boneless, skinless chicken breasts, sliced
- 2 tablespoons olive oil
- 2 cloves garlic, minced
- 2 tablespoons soy sauce
- 1 tablespoon fish sauce
- 1 tablespoon lime juice
- 1 tablespoon peanut butter
- 1 teaspoon sriracha sauce (optional)
- 2 eggs, beaten
- 1/4 cup chopped peanuts
- 2 tablespoons chopped fresh cilantro

Directions

1. Warm the olive oil in a large non-stick skillet over moderately high heat. Add minced garlic and chicken breast slices. Cook until the chicken is thoroughly cooked, approximately 5 to 6 minutes. Please take out the chicken from the pan and set it aside.
2. In the same skillet, add the zucchini noodles and cook for 2-3 minutes, until tender-crisp.
3. Whisk together the soy sauce, fish sauce, lime juice, peanut butter, and sriracha sauce in a small bowl. Pour the sauce over the zucchini noodles and toss to coat.
4. Push the zucchini noodles to one side of the skillet. Pour the beaten eggs into the space and scramble them.
5. Add the prepared chicken back to the skillet and stir to combine everything.
6. Serve the low-carb chicken Pad Thai garnished with chopped peanuts and fresh cilantro.

Nutrition Information

Calories: 280 , Total Fat: 15g , Total Carbohydrates: 10g , Fiber: 3g , Protein: 25g

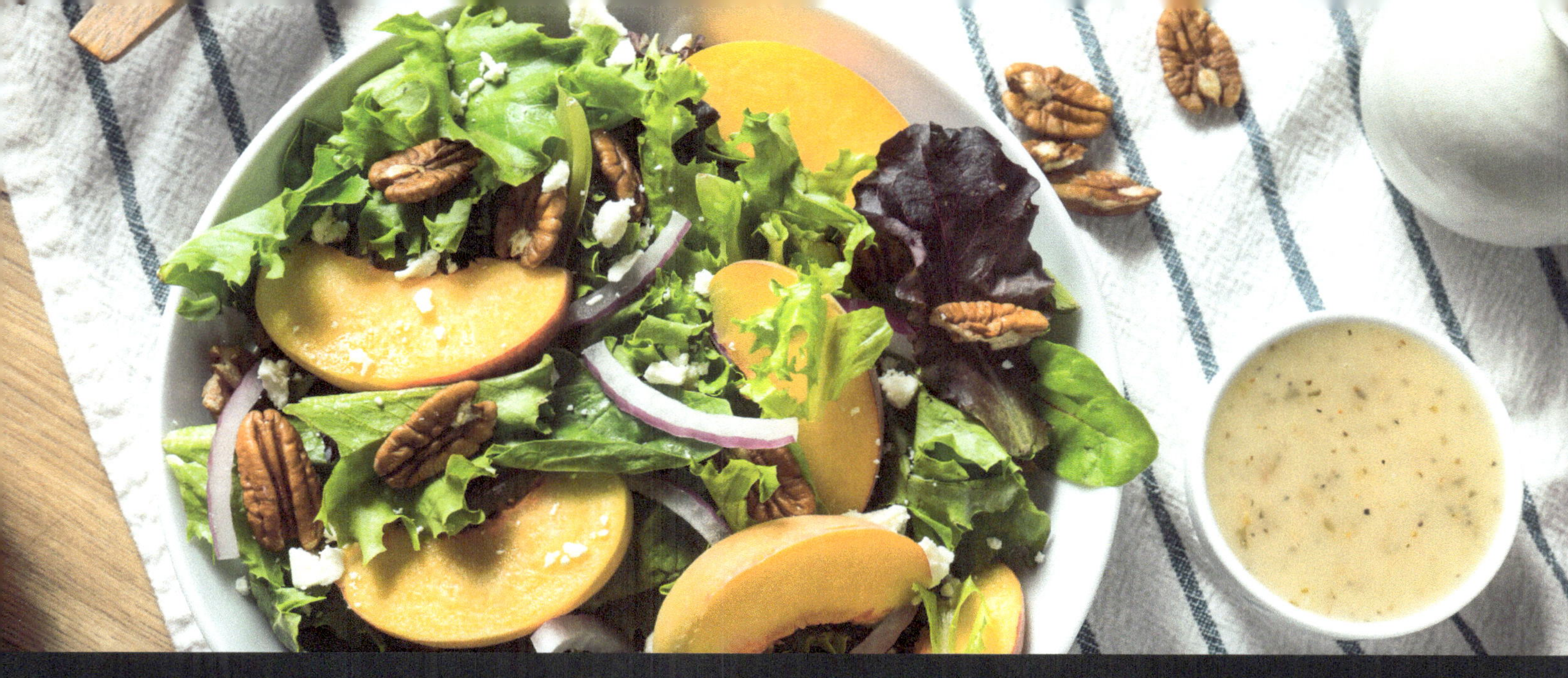

GRILLED PEACH SALAD

Preparation Time	Cooking Time	Servings
10 min	6 min	4

- 4 peaches, halved and pitted
- 4 cups mixed salad greens
- 1/2 cup crumbled feta cheese
- 1/4 cup chopped pecans
- 2 tablespoons balsamic vinegar
- 2 tablespoons olive oil
- Salt and pepper to taste

Directions

1. Preheat your grill to medium-high heat.
2. Set the peach halves on the grill, and cut the side down. Grill for 2-3 minutes until grill marks appear.
3. Combine the mixed salad greens, crumbled feta cheese, and chopped pecans in a large bowl.
4. Whisk the balsamic vinegar, olive oil, salt, and pepper in a bowl. Drizzle the dressing on the salad & toss to coat.
5. Remove the grilled peach halves from the grill and slice them.
6. Arrange the grilled peaches on top of the salad.

Nutrition Information

Calories: 180 , Total Fat: 12g , Total Carbohydrates: 15g , Fiber: 3g , Protein: 5g

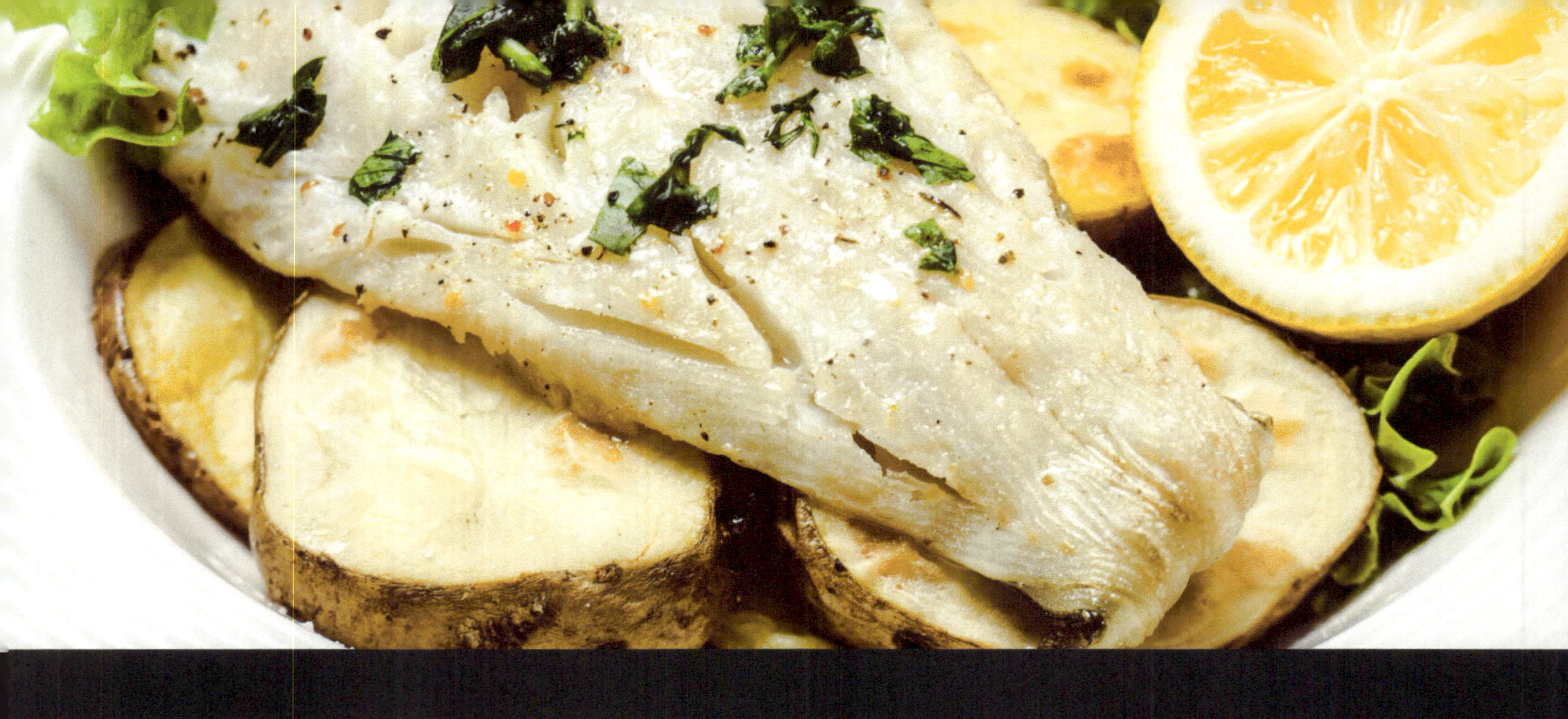

LEMON HERB COD

<table>
<tr><td>Preparation Time
10 min</td><td>Cooking Time
15 min</td><td>Servings
4</td></tr>
</table>

Ingredients

- 4 cod fillets
- 2 tablespoons olive oil
- 2 tablespoons lemon juice
- 1 tbsp chopped fresh herbs (such as parsley, dill, or thyme)
- 2 cloves garlic, minced
- Salt & pepper to taste

Directions

1. Adjust the temperature of the oven to 400°F (200°C).
2. Place fish fillets on a parchment-lined baking sheet.
3. Mix olive oil, lime juice, chopped fresh herbs, minced garlic, salt & pepper in a bowl.
4. Brush the herb blending over the cod fillets, coating evenly.
5. Set a few slices of lemon on top of each fillet.
6. Bake the cod for 12-15 minutes until opaque and fork-tender.
7. Serve the lemon herb cod with additional lemon slices on the side.

Nutrition Information

Calories: 200 , Total Fat: 9g , Total Carbohydrates: 1g , Fiber: 0g , Protein: 28g

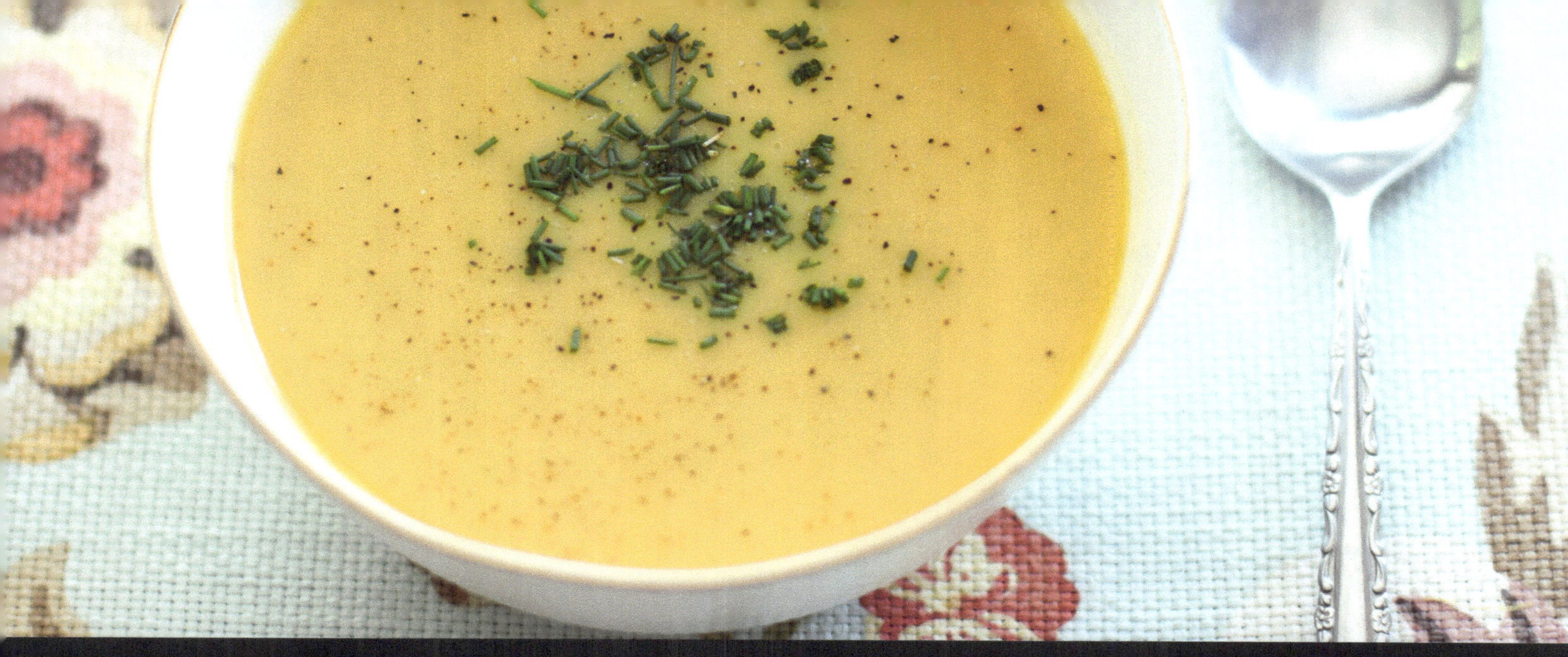

CURRIED BUTTERNUT SQUASH SOUP

Ingredients

Preparation Time	Cooking Time	Servings
15 min	30 min	4

- 1 butternut squash, peeled, seeded, and cubed
- 1 onion, chopped
- 2 cloves garlic, minced
- 2 teaspoons curry powder
- 1/2 teaspoon ground cinnamon
- 1/4 teaspoon ground nutmeg
- 4 cups vegetable broth
- 1 cup unsweetened coconut milk
- Salt and pepper to taste
- Fresh cilantro for garnish

Directions

1. Combine the cubed butternut squash, chopped onion, minced garlic, curry powder, ground cinnamon, ground nutmeg, vegetable broth, salt, and pepper in a large pot.
2. Take the mixture to a boil, then reduce heat and simmer for 20-25 minutes or until the butternut squash is tender.
3. Use an immersion blender or move the soup to puree until smooth.
4. Take the soup back to the pot and stir in the coconut milk. Heat gently until warmed through.
5. Serve the curried butternut squash soup garnished with fresh cilantro.

Nutrition Information

Calories: 180 , Total Fat: 8g , Total Carbohydrates: 29g , Fiber: 6g , Protein: 3g

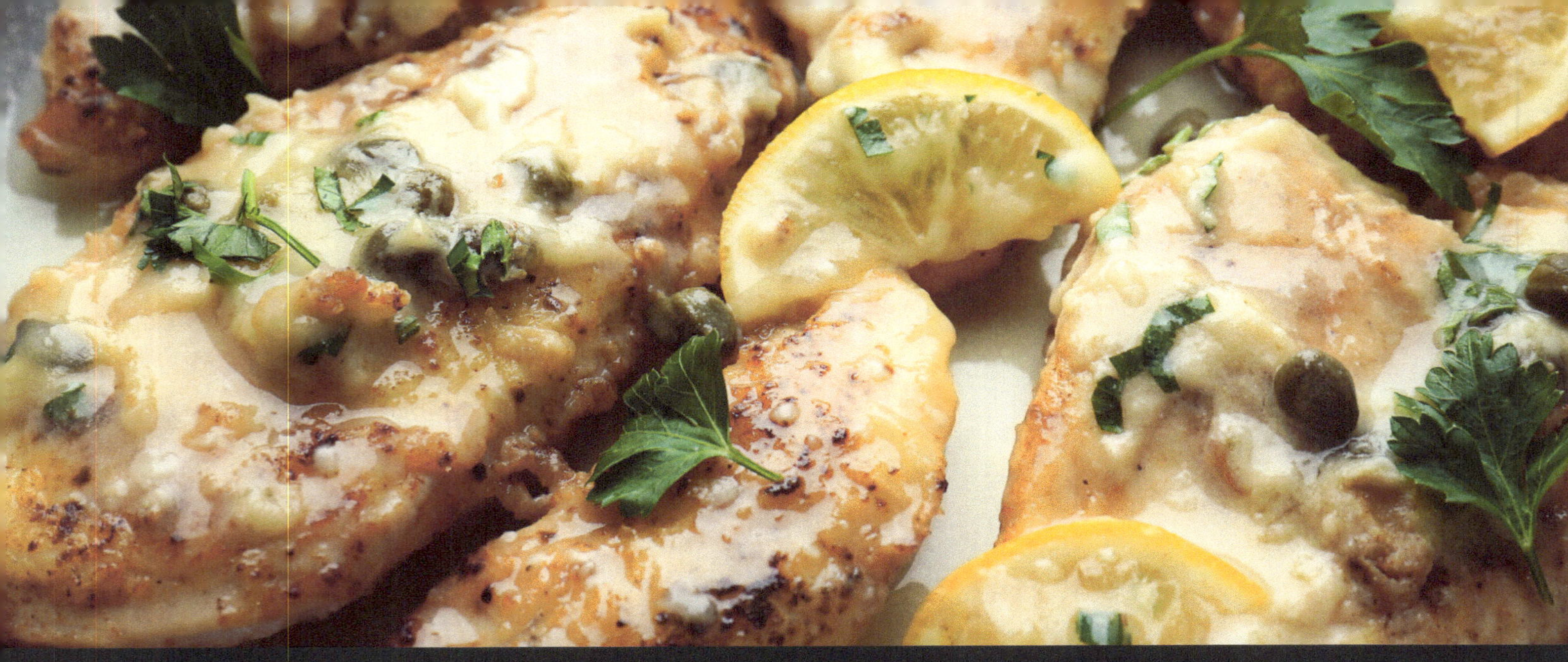

TILAPIA PICCATA

Preparation Time	Cooking Time	Servings
10 min	15 min	4

- 4 tilapia fillets
- 2 tablespoons olive oil
- 2 tablespoons butter
- 2 cloves garlic, minced
- 1/2 cup chicken broth
- 1/4 cup lemon juice
- 2 tablespoons capers
- 2 tablespoons chopped fresh parsley
- Salt and pepper to taste

Directions

1. Add salt and pepper to the tilapia pieces.
2. Large skillet, medium-high heat, olive oil, and butter. Cook garlic for 1 minute.
3. Cook the tilapia fillets in the skillet for 3-4 mins on each side until gets golden brown and cooked through. Take the fish out of the pan and set
4. it aside.
5. Add chicken broth and lime juice to the skillet. Simmer for 2 minutes, scraping the skillet to blend flavors.
6. Mix in the chopped capers and fresh parsley.
7. Pour the sauce over the tilapia fillets. Cook the sauce for 1 to 2 minutes, until it is warm.
8. Serve the tilapia piccata with the sauce spooned over the top.

Nutrition Information

Calories: 240 , Total Fat: 12g , Total Carbohydrates: 2g , Fiber: 0g , Protein: 31g

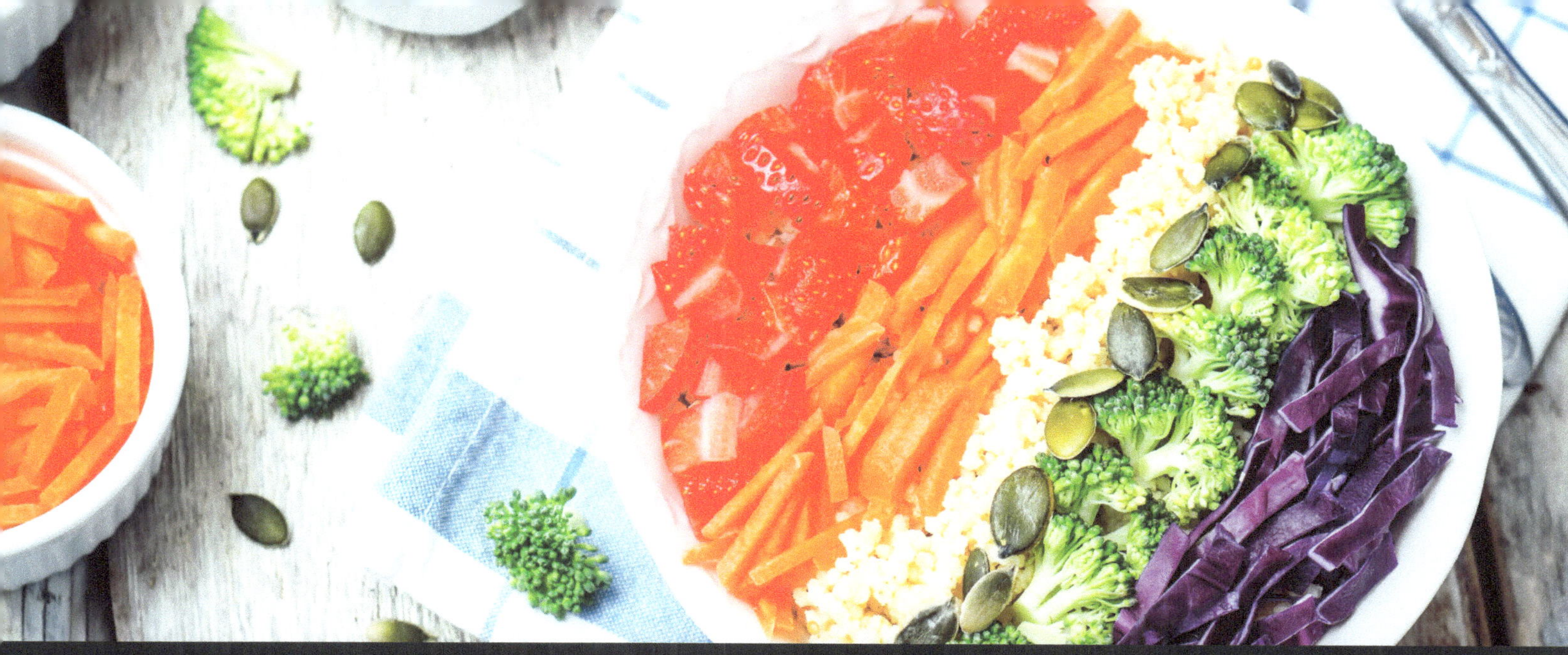

RAINBOW VEGETABLE SALAD

Preparation Time	Cooking Time	Servings
15 min	0 min	4

- 2 cups mixed salad greens
- 1 cup cherry tomatoes, halved
- 1 cup diced cucumber
- 1/2 cup sliced bell peppers (red, yellow, or orange)
- 1/2 cup shredded carrots
- 1/4 cup sliced red onion
- 2 tablespoons balsamic vinegar
- 1 tablespoon olive oil
- Salt and pepper to taste

Directions

1. Combine the mixed salad greens, cherry tomatoes, diced cucumber, sliced bell peppers, shredded carrots, and sliced red onion in a large bowl.
2. Mix the balsamic vinegar, olive oil, salt, and pepper in a small bowl with a whisk. Drizzle the dressing over the salad and swirl to distribute evenly.
3. Serve the rainbow vegetable salad as a side dish, or add grilled chicken or tofu to make it a main course.

Nutrition Information

Calories: 80 , Total Fat: 4g , Total Carbohydrates: 10g , Fiber: 3g
Protein: 2g

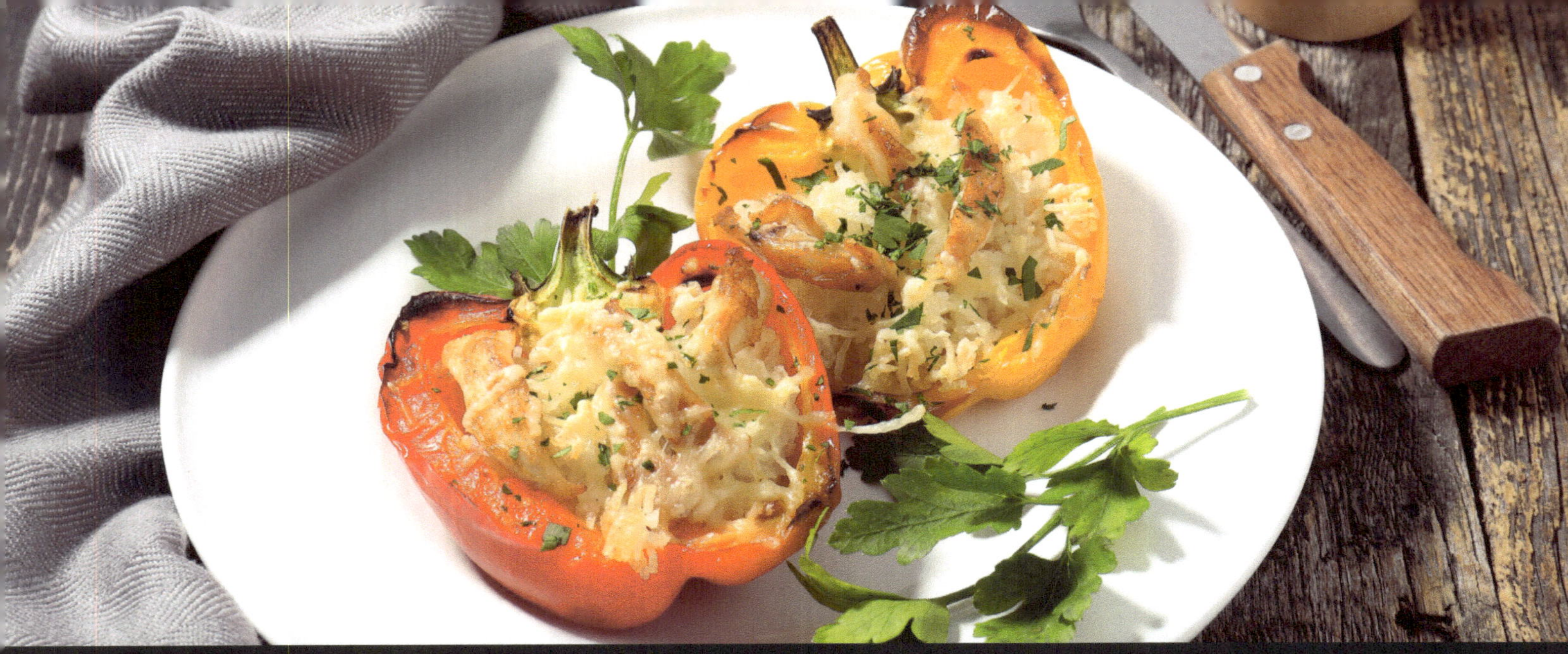

STUFFED BELL PEPPERS

Preparation Time	Cooking Time	Servings
20 min	40 min	4

- 4 bell peppers (any color)
- 1 tablespoon olive oil
- 1/2 cup diced onion
- 2 cloves garlic, minced
- 1 lb. ground turkey
- 1 cup cooked quinoa
- 1 can diced tomatoes
- 1 teaspoon dried oregano
- 1 teaspoon dried basil
- Salt and pepper to taste
- Shredded cheese for topping (optional)

Directions

1. Prepare a temperature in your oven of 375°F (190 degrees Celsius).
2. Remove bell pepper seeds and membranes.
3. Heat olive oil in a big skillet on medium. Add onion and garlic. About 5 minutes.
4. Add the ground turkey or lean beef to the skillet and cook until browned. Drain any excess fat.
5. Stir in the cooked quinoa, diced tomatoes, dried oregano, dried basil, salt, and pepper. Cook for an additional 5 minutes until heated through.
6. Fill each bell pepper with the turkey or beef mixture. Set the stuffed peppers in a baking dish.
7. Bake in the oven for 30-35 mins or until the bell peppers are tender.
8. If desired, sprinkle shredded cheese on top of each stuffed pepper during the last 5 minutes of baking.

Calories: 300 , Total Fat: 10g , Total Carbohydrates: 28g , Fiber: 6g , Protein: 250

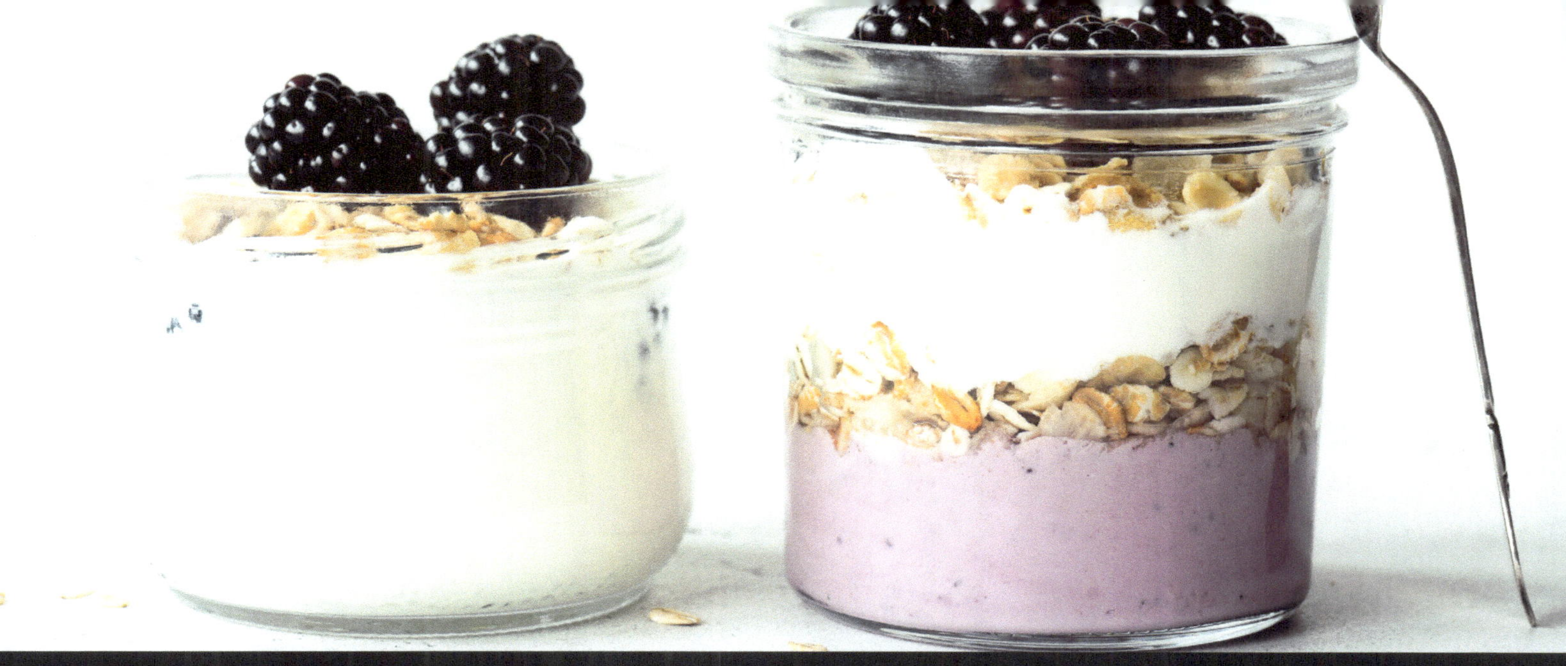

GREEK YOGURT PARFAIT

Preparation Time	Cooking Time	Servings
5 min	0 min	1

- 1/2 cup Greek yogurt
- 1/4 cup granola
- 1/4 cup fresh berries (such as strawberries, blueberries, or raspberries)
- 1 tablespoon honey or maple syrup (optional)
- 1 tablespoon chopped nuts (such as almonds or walnuts) (optional)

Directions

1. Layer the Greek yogurt, granola, and fresh berries in a glass jar.
2. Drizzle with honey or maple syrup if desired.
3. Sprinkle with chopped nuts if desired.
4. Repeat the layers if making multiple servings.
5. Serve the Greek yogurt parfait immediately or refrigerate for later.

Nutrition Information

Calories: 200 , Total Fat: 6g , Total Carbohydrates: 30g , Fiber: 4g , Protein: 10g

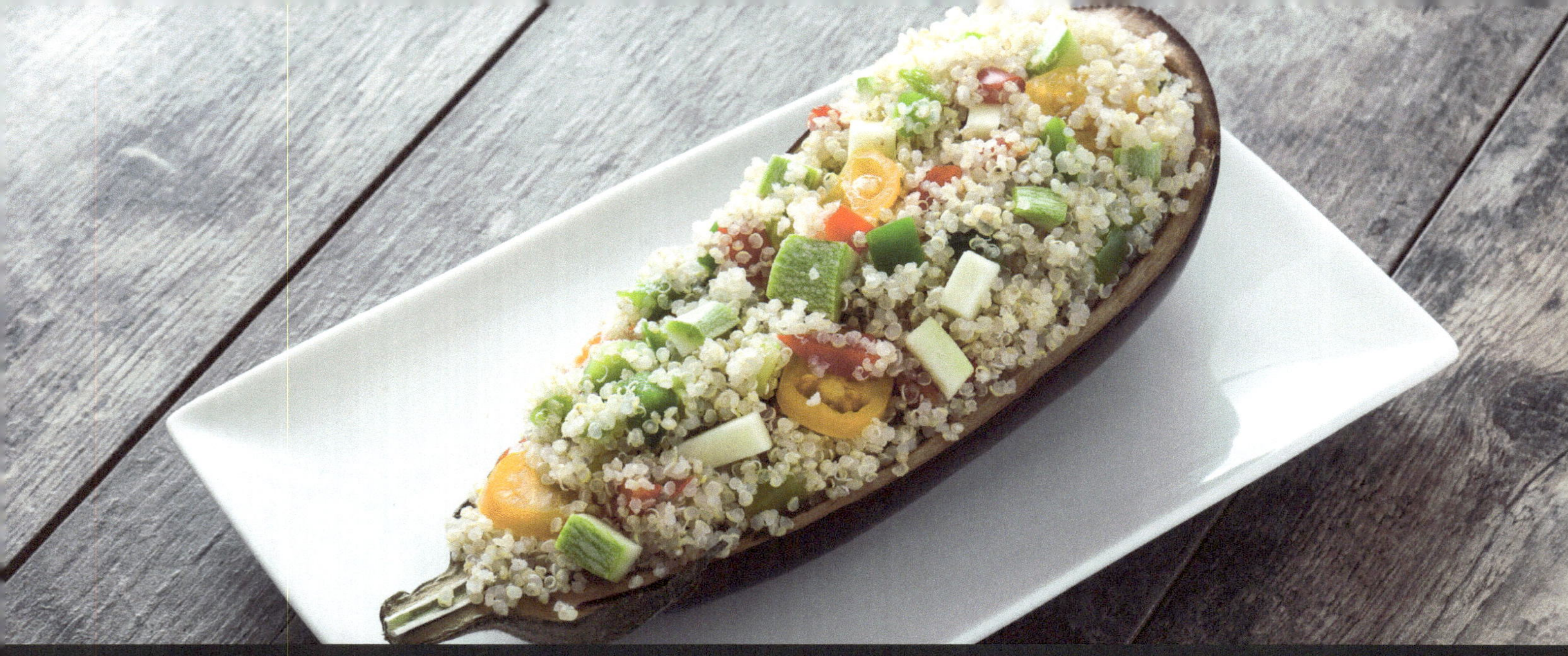

QUINOA STUFFED EGGPLANT

<table>
<tr><th>Preparation Time
15 min</th><th>Cooking Time
40 min</th><th>Servings
4</th></tr>
</table>

Ingredients

- 2 large eggplants
- 1 cup cooked quinoa
- 1/2 cup diced onion
- 2 cloves garlic, minced
- 1/2 cup diced tomatoes
- 1/4 cup chopped fresh parsley
- 2 tablespoons grated Parmesan cheese
- 1 tablespoon olive oil
- Salt and pepper to taste

Directions

1. Adjust your oven to 375°F (190°C).
2. Cut the eggplants in half lengthwise. Scoop out the flesh, leaving a 1/4-inch thick shell.
3. Chop the eggplant flesh into small pieces.
4. In a large non-stick skillet, heat the olive oil over moderate heat. Add the diced onion, minced garlic, and chopped eggplant flesh. Prepare until the onion is translucent and the eggplant is tender, about 5 minutes.
5. Stir in the cooked quinoa, diced tomatoes, chopped fresh parsley, grated Parmesan cheese, salt, and pepper. Cook for an additional 2-3 mins until heated through.
6. Spoon the quinoa mixture into the eggplant shells, dividing it evenly.
7. Set the stuffed eggplants in a baking dish and cover with foil.
8. Prepare in the oven for 30-35 mins or until the eggplants are tender.

Nutrition Information

Calories: 180, Total Fat: 6g , Total Carbohydrates: 27g , Fiber: 8g , Protein: 6g

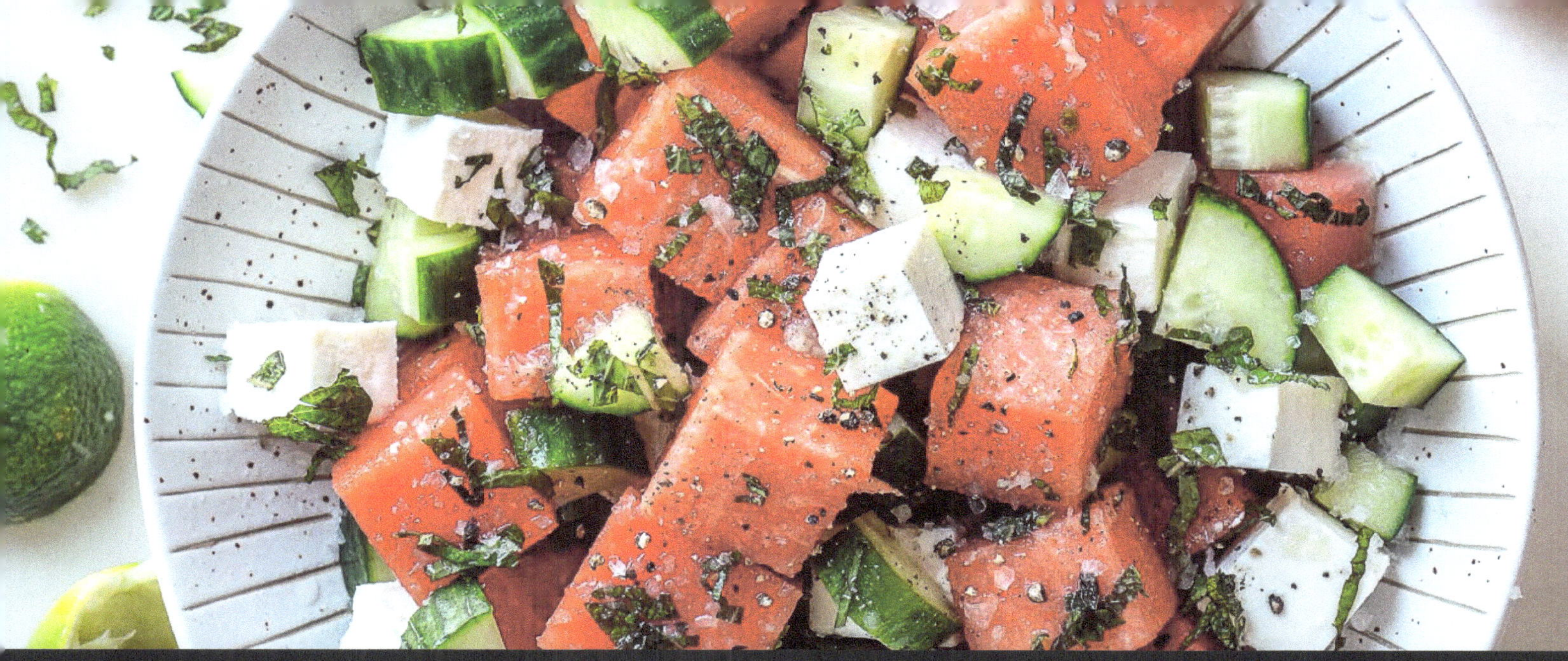

WATERMELON CUCUMBER FETA SALAD

Preparation Time	Cooking Time	Servings
10 min	0 min	6

Ingredients

- 6 cups watermelon, seeded and cubed
- 1 English cucumber, chopped
- 6 oz feta cheese, cubed
- a handful of chopped fresh mint leaves
- 1 fresh lime, zest and juice
- sea salt flakes and fresh ground black pepper, to taste

Directions

1. Add your cubed watermelon into a large serving bowl along with the rest of your ingredients.
2. Very gently toss to combine.
3. Taste test, and adjust if desired.
4. Serve and enjoy!

Nutrition Information

Calories: 120, Total Fat: 6g , Total Carbohydrates: 14g , Fiber: 1g , Protein: 4g